Her-2

Her-2

The Making of Herceptin,
a Revolutionary Treatment
for Breast Cancer

ROBERT BAZELL

With an Introduction
by Dr. Mary-Claire King

RANDOM HOUSE / NEW YORK

To Margot, Rebecca, Josh, and Stephanie

*And to the memory of Rebecca Donovan who
taught us the terror of this disease
and courage in the face of it*

CONTENTS

ACKNOWLEDGMENTS

My greatest debt is to the people who took the time to educate me about the many facets of this story—especially the remarkable women with advanced breast cancer, the volunteers for the clinical trials, who shared so much of their own experience. To them and to all the others listed in the Notes at the end, my profound thanks for the time spent, especially for seemingly endless follow-up phone calls and e-mails to which I subjected some.

I want to thank Laura Leber of Genentech for facilitating my access to the many people in the company who were willing to talk with me and for responding to my many inquiries, always with patient, good cheer. John Dreyfuss played a similar, wonderfully helpful role at UCLA's Jonsson Cancer Center.

Ann Godoff, now editor in chief and president of Random House, persuaded me to write this book and managed to continue to serve as its editor while she took on all the management responsibilities. I remain in awe. Suzanne Gluck of ICM not only educated me about the need for a book agent but also taught me how the very best in the trade do it. Amy Bernstein provided invaluable assistance with the writing and editing, as did Ruth Coughlin. My special thanks to Carolyn Schatz, my colleague and good friend of sixteen years, without whose research and writing assistance this project simply could not have happened.

My profound gratitude also to the following people who were kind enough to read this manuscript or portions of it during its various stages of development: Josh Bazell, Hank Fuchs, V. Craig Jordan, Al Rabson, Betty Rollin, Lynn Schuchter, Robert Weinberg, Margot Weinshel, and J. Frank Wilson. Their suggestions helped me greatly, but of course I alone am responsible for all the opinions expressed and any errors that might have been made.

INTRODUCTION

by Dr. Mary-Claire King
American Cancer Society professor of genetics,
University of Washington

After the British victory at the Battle of El Alamein in 1942, Winston Churchill said, "Now this is not the end. It is not even the beginning of the end. But it is, perhaps, the end of the beginning."

He was, of course, correct. Churchill's elegant language speaks to many of us who are involved in an entirely different kind of war, the one against the multiheaded, insidious, and complex destruction of normal cellular life that is cancer. This is the story of an important and early victory in that war.

The "war on cancer" was declared in 1971 by Richard Nixon, the unlikeliest of heroes to many of us who grew up in the 1960s, protesting another war. But in putting enormous public resources into cancer research, Nixon turned out to be prescient. For this war on cancer, the strategy was intelligent, albeit unfaithful to the military analogy that had spawned it. In its dependence on individual investigators who were sought out for their keen tactics and for their willingness to take risks, the war was more guerrilla than top-down strategy. To continue the analogy, it was more American Revolution than Vietnam.

"The end of the beginning": The story told herein starts with the identification by Robert Weinberg in 1979 of "HER-2/neu," a gene involved in multiple cancer pathways. Years of more hard work would reveal that Her-2/neu could be a target for a new type of breast cancer treatment.

Why is it that twenty-seven years into the war we are only now declaring the first victory—the "end of the beginning"? Elegant biology often seems obvious after the fact. Vast collections of ideas were spawned by the war on cancer—many of them very good, some so good as to be perceived as hopelessly risky. During its early life, the HER-2 project was ridiculed, close to impossible to fund, and nearly abandoned more than once.

The translation of this now-obvious biology into drug development and cancer treatment is a drama too good to be fiction. It is uniquely a story of the late twentieth century, and its heroes are peculiarly American: stubborn and straightforward, they can be seen as mavericks, cowboys, lone rangers. The first of these are the scientists: Dennis Slamon, a UCLA oncologist and cell biologist, the son of a coal miner and grandson of a Syrian immigrant; and Axel Ullrich, one of the first gene cloners, who moved from Germany to California and joined the biotechnology company Genentech in its early days. Between them, Slamon and Ullrich discovered the critical role of HER-2/neu in breast-cancer development.

To create a drug based on this biology required a great deal of rigorous immunology, largely carried out by scientists at Genentech. Although these scientists were personally committed to the project, it encountered labyrinthine vicissitudes at the hands of a corporate culture that was concerned with the firm's sheer survival. Happily, and certainly not easily, a few people with talent in both science and management emerged from this maelstrom.

The other heroes in this tale are the breast-cancer patients and their partners. It is difficult to imagine a more moving love story than the effective tribute of Bob Erwin to his wife, Marti Nelson, a physician who died at the age of forty from metastatic breast cancer before she could be treated with the antibody. Erwin, along with activists in San Francisco who took their cues from AIDS activists, focused on bringing together Genentech management and breast-cancer advocates into a working alliance. Armed with this knowledge of biology and biotechnology management and propelled by grief over his wife's death, Erwin pushed and persuaded and persevered to establish compassionate use of the antibody.

The expense of proving the usefulness of a drug in phase III trials is daunting. Because the appropriate patients were being treated in many widely dispersed hospitals and because many of their physicians had no previous experience with this sort of trial, putting it together was a logistical nightmare.

Enter Fran Visco—lawyer, consumer advocate, breast-cancer survivor, and, as chairwoman of the National Breast Cancer Coalition, an extraordinarily competent organizer. Visco learned the science, decided that the NBCC should support the test, and sent information about the trials to thousands of patients and physicians, paving the way for hundreds of women to sign up.

The phase III trial results, revealed in spring 1998, did indeed prove that Herceptin worked as well as anyone dared hope. Because of this, perhaps fifty thousand breast-cancer patients a year will benefit. As Dennis Slamon has said, "This is proof of the principle that we can identify what's broken in a cancer cell and fix it."

This, then, is a fable for our time. It is one with many tragic losses and an ultimately happy ending, or at least one that is hopeful. It is a complex biological mystery; a drama of high finance; a series of nonsentimental, intelligent love stories; and a terrific vindication of stubbornness in a good cause.

In all, it proves that good science makes a great yarn.

PROLOGUE

Dennis Slamon felt his heart pounding. For years, the six-foot-two, robust doctor with the distinctive mustache had fantasized about this moment, but never had he imagined himself so nervous.

Approaching fifty, Slamon had spent much of his career, thirteen years in fact, obsessed with a molecule called Her-2. A genetic mutation prompts Her-2 to flourish in excess in some breast cancer. Slamon believed Her-2 held the key to nothing less than curing breast cancer, not all breast cancer, but a significant amount of it. With murderous resolve, Slamon had sought to prove that belief. Now he was prepared to offer the evidence—details of a study of a drug called Herceptin that homed in on Her-2 to obliterate breast-cancer cells. The occasion was the annual gathering of his peers.

The American Society for Clinical Oncology (ASCO), the professional organization of cancer specialists, meets in a different city every year. In May 1998, the doctors assembled in the Los Angeles Convention Center, a steel and glass monstrosity situated in a deserted section of the city's downtown.

For most of the convention, oncologists shuffle from session to session, carrying bags stuffed with coffee mugs, clocks, notepads, and other gifts, all emblazoned with logos of drug companies and their cancer medications, picked up at the gaudy display booths in the commercial exhibit halls. The doctors hear about seemingly endless studies of treatments for all forms of cancer, but seldom does any one treatment translate into better patient survival. In fact, so little genuine progress occurs in the fight against cancer that a dark joke circulating among the doctors had it that more cancer patients would be saved if a bomb went off, demolishing the convention center and all the oncologists with it.

But on Sunday afternoon, May 17, most of the eighteen thousand delegates passed up an opportunity to enjoy the bright sunshine outside and instead crowded into the convention center's dim and cavernous West Hall. In anticipatory silence, they waited for Slamon, director of the Revlon/UCLA Women's Cancer Research Program, to ascend the podium. His talk, they expected, would detail this entirely new weapon against a very common cancer.

At a press conference earlier that morning, Craig Henderson, a well-known breast-cancer specialist, had described Herceptin as "the first step in the future," a gene-based treatment that moves away from the "poisons" that had dominated cancer treatment. He declared that the investment in the War on Cancer that President Nixon had declared back in 1971 was finally paying off. "It's like the taxpayers are getting their money back for the first time," he said. "This is science at its most elegant and best."

In the weeks before the convention, a sort of hysteria about cancer treatment had gripped the country. It began with an article that appeared on the front page of the Sunday, May 3, 1998 *New York Times* ("A Cautious Awe Greets Drugs That Eradicate Tumors in Mice") suggesting that cancer—all cancer—could be cured in two years. The miracle cure, the article implied, was a combination of two drugs, angiostatin and endostatin, that appear to choke off the blood supply to tumors, preventing them from growing and spreading. Buried in the story was the fact that the new drugs had not yet been tested in human beings. In effect, the article was cruel hype that led thousands of desperate patients to call doctors and hospitals begging for these new drugs that did not yet exist in any form suitable for human use. Angiostatin, endostatin, and other anti-angiogenesis drugs, as they are known, may prove someday to be effective. But years of human tests stand between hope and reality. In marked contrast, Dennis Slamon was about to tell this gathering of oncologists about Herceptin, a drug that already had been tested in hundreds of breast cancer patients. It would be on the market, available to women with breast cancer, in the fall of 1998, only a few months away.

To be sure, Herceptin did not cure all breast cancer. It had the potential to treat an extraordinarily aggressive and intractable form of the disease that accounts for 25 to 30 percent of cases. Women with that form of breast cancer often face terrible prognoses, their cancers recurring a few months to a few years after diagnosis. Herceptin improved and prolonged the lives of these women—in some cases effecting what looked like a cure. The drug did not always work. Slamon and others were struggling to learn why. Nevertheless, what made Herceptin deserve such adjectives as "revolutionary" and "breakthrough," what made it stand out from previous cancer treatments, was that it targeted cancer cells specifically without damaging normal tissue. Because of that precision, the new treatment did not bring the hair loss, nausea, anemia, or the other dreaded side effects that so often accompany cancer treatments.

Scientists had been predicting such targeted, laboratory-designed cancer treatments for decades—so many years, in fact, that much of the public and medical profession had assumed it would never happen. But Slamon was now offering data from an eloquent clinical trial. Surely more scientifically targeted treatments would follow. Other studies presented at the same meeting detailed dozens of such promising drugs at earlier stages of testing. But the first one—Herceptin—had arrived.

Little of great scientific and medical significance is achieved without exhausting effort. But Slamon perceived his campaign to bestow the new breast-cancer drug on patients as an unending battle against nearly overwhelming forces of opposition. Many of his colleagues, academic oncologists sitting in the audience this very afternoon, had ridiculed both him and his ideas. Most often, they portrayed him as a man hopelessly obsessed with a single idea that would never work. Few had shown up to listen to his sessions at past ASCO meetings. Everyone claimed to want a better breast-cancer treatment, but when a potential one came along, prejudices about treatment options kept many oncologists from giving it much consideration. Until recently Slamon had enjoyed little collegial encouragement.

As an academic physician, Slamon could not bring a drug to market. Only a corporation can muster the enormous necessary resources. Genentech, the biotechnology company based in South San Francisco, owned the rights to Herceptin. But Genentech's involvement had its price. Several times the company had tried to quash the project, motivated, Slamon thought, by indecision, shortsighted business considerations, and simple mistakes. But now Genentech, which had spent an estimated $200 million and an enormous amount of time on Herceptin, seemed to regard Herceptin as a great victory, *its* great victory, not Dennis Slamon's. Just as Slamon believed he was attaining the success he had sought for so long, he sensed that Genentech was trying hard to rewrite the history of the project, obliterating the crucial role he had played. In addition, some of the same doctors who had ridiculed the work at its earlier stages were making moves to swallow it and spit it out as their own.

Struggle was hardly unfamiliar to Slamon. Having grown up in a family so poor that the local Boy Scout troop and neighboring families donated groceries to keep young Dennis and his parents from starving, he was no stranger to tests of endurance. Scholarships enabled him to escape to the world of academic medicine, and once there he managed to ascend to a perch far above the typical medical school professor. A chance encounter with a single patient opened a floodgate of money for his research efforts from the Revlon corporation. With the funding, he achieved not only power in his academic life but also access to the glamour of Hollywood and wealthy New York society.

Two days before his appearance at ASCO, the front page of the Marketplace section of *The Wall Street Journal* featured a large cartoon of Slamon with supermodels Cindy Crawford and Halle Berry on either arm. Models and other celebrities often visited Slamon's lab to help publicize the Revlon contribution. That article and other publicity generated no small amount of snickering and obvious jealousy from some other oncologists. One of the country's best-known breast cancer specialists, Larry Norton of Memorial Sloan Kettering in New York, was incredulous, rolling his eyes as he asked one friend after another at the meeting if they had seen the *Journal* article. "It's as if Denny Slamon developed Herceptin all by himself," Norton commented. But Slamon believed that he *did* do it by himself, or almost.

His image projected on two twenty-five-foot-tall television screens, Dennis Slamon ascended to the podium to begin his presentation. A certain tightness had taken over his features, an expression that could even be construed as a grimace. He started out not by describing the results of Herceptin's groundbreaking clinical trial, but by offering a history lesson to set the record straight about the origins and development of this revolutionary drug.

After he concluded his talk, Slamon thanked many people. But his most impassioned gratitude was reserved for the hundreds of women, breast cancer patients, who had volunteered for this extraordinarily complicated clinical trial, the results of which were about to propel Herceptin into the marketplace, ushering in a wholly new era of cancer treatment.

Her-2

Discovering Cancer

One morning in the fall of 1978, Anne McNamara showered while her husband, Jeff, tended to Luke, their one-year-old son. As she soaped and scrubbed, she felt something unfamiliar in her left breast. "Uh-oh," she thought, a chill going down her spine. She had a history of fibrocystic disease. She tried to convince herself that all this could be was just another benign growth. Silently she recited the statistics: she was thirty-two; in premenopausal women, just one out of twelve tumors turns out to be cancerous. Fighting the impulse to panic, she sought comfort in the knowledge that there was no history of cancer in her family.

Anne McNamara brought uncommon understanding to her discovery. Having been a biology major and a chemistry minor in college, her first job had been in a laboratory of a scientist at Yale Medical School, who was carrying out medical research. She tested the effects of radiation and chemotherapy on cancer cells. Much as she wanted to believe that this lump, like many others she had previously had, would go away as she moved through her monthly hormonal cycle, she had a feeling that this one was different. In unguarded moments over the next couple of weeks, she probed the new growth. Had it changed? Did it feel different? Once you find a lump, she says, "You check it three times a day." After more than a month had passed without any change in the lump, she went to see her gynecologist, who said he thought it was just a cyst. Nonetheless, he sent her to a surgeon for a biopsy. Just to be sure.

A few days later, McNamara met with her doctor, James Finn, who offered her the choice that most women in her position then faced: he could do the biopsy and wait until McNamara came out of the anesthesia to give her the results, or they could agree ahead of time that he would remove her breast if the tumor turned out to be malignant. McNamara, typically matter-of-fact, chose the second option, the course of least emotional complication. As Jeff remembers it, "She did not fear the worst, but she prepared for the worst."

Anne's delicate appearance and honeyed Georgia accent belie her toughness. Her face settles naturally into a warm smile, and when she talks in her straightforward and low-key manner, her large green eyes and her high-arched eyebrows give the listener a clear window on her emotions. She's now a youthful fifty-two years old, with auburn hair flowing to her shoulders. Jeff, a muscular man with a neatly trimmed mustache and ice-blue eyes, had just returned from a four-year stint in the Air Force and was finishing up his business degree when they met. They lived in the same apartment building in New Haven; when Anne had totaled her motorcycle, and Jeff, an inveterate tinkerer, saw it crumpled in a corner of the garage, he asked her if he could take a crack at fixing it. They've been together ever since.

Anne's surgery was scheduled for the week after Thanksgiving. Jeff stayed home with the baby and awaited word from the hospital. In the operating room, the surgeon was stunned by the lump's size: five centimeters, the size of a lemon. Moments later, a pathologist confirmed that it was a tumor and it was indeed malignant. Dr. Jim (as the McNamaras called him) phoned Jeff from the operat-

ing room. "It's not good, Jeff." "How not good?" "Bad." Jeff paused
to collect himself and then said, "Do what you've got to do. Take
care of her the best way that you know how."

McNamara remembers slowly coming out of the anesthesia. "I
was still extremely groggy, and I was trying to figure out if my
breast was gone or not. I knew if it was, then it meant I had cancer.
But I was so groggy that I clutched at my chest and I couldn't figure it out." As the anesthesia wore off, she realized that her torso
was wrapped in a bandage. "I knew what that meant."

Her doctor was flabbergasted. "We were all flabbergasted," said
McNamara. "Because it *was* cancer, and there I was, thirty-two
years old, although now it's getting more and more common to
happen in younger and younger women. But in 1978 it was still unusual enough that the doctor just couldn't believe it. Who knows
where it came from? But it had probably been there seven or eight
years by that time, they say, before you can feel anything."

In 1978, the initial treatment of breast cancer had not changed
much since the end of the nineteenth century. Like Anne McNamara, most women undergoing surgical biopsy would drift off into
the oblivion of anesthesia and grab at their chests when they awoke
to learn whether they had lost a breast or not. When McNamara
underwent surgery, enlightened doctors still considered the radical
mastectomy, a decades-old procedure, the best choice for cases like
hers.

McNamara's first question on learning that she had cancer was
whether she needed chemotherapy. Even though she knew all
about the side effects, like nausea and hair loss, she thought it
might help keep the cancer at bay. But Dr. Jim tried to assure her
that he had gotten all traces of the disease and recommended
against it. McNamara felt relieved, but suspicious. "I remember
thinking to myself, 'He doesn't really know that,' " she says. She
spent enough time around cancer research to know that rogue cancer cells often escape to other parts of the body before surgery.

Why not have chemotherapy as insurance against spread or recurrence? Dr. Jim argued that chemotherapy could actually spur cancer to recur and cited very preliminary Russian studies on premenopausal women that purported to show how chemotherapy could actually induce the spread of breast cancer. Those studies were soon discredited, but they illustrated a truth about medicine: state-of-the-art practices come and go as medical science proves and then discredits its latest thinking. Even the most immaculately reasoned advice can be faulty.

In fact, by the time Anne McNamara had her mastectomy, clinical trials were already under way that would prove the usefulness of chemotherapy immediately after breast-cancer surgery. McNamara did not care about trends in cancer treatment; she only wanted to take every precaution against her disease, and her instincts told her that chemotherapy would increase the chances of eradicating her cancer. While disheartened, she did not challenge Dr. Jim. As happens so often, the patient was protecting the caregiver. "He was trying to comfort me, and he was a friend." Thinking back on it now, McNamara wonders if chemotherapy might have saved her from the terror of recurring cancer. Then she dismisses the thought: "That was the accepted protocol at the time."

McNamara's instincts turned out to be better than her surgeon's. Ten years after her mastectomy, the National Cancer Institute issued an emergency clinical alert to physicians, recommending that chemotherapy follow soon after surgery for all but the least threatening breast-cancer cases. Clinical trials had demonstrated convincingly that chemotherapy administered right after cancer surgery—called adjuvant chemotherapy—could help prevent the disease from returning and could thus improve the patient's chances of survival. Nowadays, adjuvant therapy is the standard of care for most breast-cancer patients.

McNamara had good reason to be so cautious. Breast cancer in a thirty-two-year-old woman is extremely rare and especially frightening. For reasons no one clearly understands, when the disease occurs so early in life, it tends to grow aggressively. In the United States, the chance that a thirty-two-year-old woman will be diagnosed with breast cancer is less than one in four thousand. Only 6 percent of breast cancers in the United States strike women under the age of forty. The odds only grow worse as women age; the chance that an eighty-five-year-old woman will have developed breast cancer over the course of her lifetime is one in eight. In McNamara's case, the only relatively good news was that tests showed that the cancer had not yet spread to her lymph nodes, meaning that the chances of a recurrence were less than they would otherwise have been.

Though half of all women with breast cancer never suffer a recurrence after the initial treatment, they are still sentenced to a life of uncertainty, never sure if they will join the half that does have a recurrence; and when the cancer reappears, it is always deadlier than it was the first time around. For Anne and Jeff, breast cancer brought a particularly severe disappointment: Luke would have to be their only child. Female hormones can fuel the growth of breast-cancer cells, so a pregnancy, with its massive hormone surges, can greatly accelerate a recurrence, especially if diseased cells have managed to escape the surgeon's knife. Nowadays doctors will allow some breast-cancer survivors to risk a pregnancy, but when Anne was diagnosed it was out of the question. "That was a blow," says Anne. "We had waited for seven years after we got married to have Luke." With her hands folded calmly in her lap, she explains, "I knew it would be silly to have another infant if there was a chance I wouldn't be around to raise it. I didn't want to leave my husband with a new baby, and I didn't want to leave a new baby without a mother."

With her knowledge from the cancer lab, Anne could interpret the facts. Jeff had no similar understanding to temper his fear. He only knew that Anne might not always be there, and even twenty years later he is visibly upset at the thought, and he speaks freely about his confusion, fear, and frustration. His take-charge attitude had worked for him during his four years in the Air Force, and it had brought him success as a consultant to high-tech companies. But here was a problem that he couldn't solve. "If it had been a hole in the roof, I could have fixed it. But there wasn't anything I could do but be around to keep our life together. I just couldn't do much else."

"I mean, I was upset," he continues. "Not traumatized, but certainly upset. But Annie puts on a very good face, and is not an outwardly worrying type. And I think that has a lot to do with it." He pauses to laugh. "I mean, she's got a steel backbone."

McNamara left the hospital a week after her mastectomy, but she still faced reconstructive surgery. Her surgeon had recommended that she not have it immediately, so she waited nearly a year. "[He] said, 'Don't do it right at first because even months afterward, whatever reconstruction you have done, it's never going to look like a real breast. It's just not the same.'" She smiles wryly when she remembers the rest of their conversation: "He said, 'If you wait a while, then when you have it, you will be so glad to have a breast again that you won't be so picky that it doesn't really look like the other one.'" She pauses while the listener savors the full arrogance of that advice. McNamara is loath to launch an attack on her doctor for his clumsy statement. She simply dismisses his comment as "a male point of view."

Waiting for reconstruction was the hard part. "I didn't feel feminine. I didn't want to have to worry with the stupid prosthesis; I wanted to be able to go swimming and wear a bathing suit and not have to worry about the dumb thing."

In the meantime, she was determined to return to her life. A computer programmer since just after her marriage, she had taken a leave of absence to care for Luke full-time. She gave whatever time she had left over to her gardening and community work. She exercised as the surgeon prescribed and recovered full use of her left arm, which had been somewhat incapacitated by the surgery. "I put cancer out of my mind," she says.

McNamara is a modest woman who is reluctant to talk about herself. She maintains a quiet reserve and regards her misfortune as her own business, never telling people about treatment except for some very good friends. She says that many people, not those to whom she felt close, just don't know what to say. "It scares them. Yes, it terrifies people, especially breast cancer, and other women particularly. And because they don't know what to say, they don't treat you like a normal person. I don't want to talk about it with casual friends. I want them to invite me over and not have the topic of conversation be illness. Oh, how *are* you, isn't it awful? How do you *feel*? You look so *pale*." But others did not share her sense of discretion.

"Word got out," she says. Friends were stunned, particularly because she was so young. When she ran errands in downtown Branford, Connecticut, mere acquaintances would race across the street to say, "I just heard the most unbelievable thing. It can't be true!" The attention and sometimes tactless concern embarrassed her. "It affected me so," she says softly. "Once people know you have cancer, that's all they remember about you. They don't know what to say, and they avoid the situation. They don't mean to, but they write you off." She stops for a moment and then adds, "I just wanted to be treated like a normal person with a future."

There were some oddly funny moments, too. She describes how some friends would glance down at her chest as they were trying to figure out which breast was real and which had been reconstructed. "They just couldn't help themselves," she chuckles. After the initial burst of concern, people began to lay off the subject. And for a while, she *was* able to put cancer out of her mind.

Until this century, cancer was considered mostly a woman's disease, and it often carried the stigma of shame. Without modern diagnostic tools, physicians could more easily recognize cancers of the breast, cervix, and ovaries. Untreated breast tumors bulge and can break through the skin; untreated cervical and ovarian cancers lead to prodigious bleeding. Thus physicians believed erroneously that cancer strikes women more often than men. Until the last twenty years or so, cancer, and most especially cancer of the female organs, was not a topic of polite conversation. In the atmosphere of denial, women were all too often left to suffer with their illness alone, unable to find support as the disease destroyed them physically and emotionally.

When Anne McNamara's breast cancer struck, the shame associated with the disease was diminishing. Since the turn of the century, improved diagnostic techniques were proving cancer to be an equal-opportunity disease. But treatment for breast cancer has improved little over the last several decades, remaining a variation on the themes of surgery, radiation, chemotherapy, and hormone treatment. Separately and in combination, these options can be effective treatments and can sometimes bring about a remission that lasts long enough to be reasonably called a cure.

Surgery does not always excise the cancer entirely. Chemotherapy and radiation are often just random attacks on the problem, destroying much but not necessarily all of the cancer and usually harming healthy tissue in the process. Hormone treatment works for some breast cancer. The new approaches, such as adjuvant chemotherapy, can bring profound benefits, but they amount to little more than adjustments to the standard procedure. The problem is that breast cancer is unpredictable. Sometimes it is wholly contained in a tumor. But all too often it spreads from the tiniest tumor long before it can be detected or removed. Why do some cancers produce micrometastases, tiny bits of cancer that migrate from the original mass? No one knows.

The death rate for breast cancer stands as a dismal monument to ignorance. It has changed little in half a century. Every year the disease strikes more than 180,000 women in the United States and kills about 44,000. In 1950, the first year the government kept such records, 264 out of every 1 million white American women died of breast cancer. Twenty-five years later, that death rate was exactly the same. By 1985, it had risen to 275. In the 1990s, it began falling slightly; by 1995 the rate had dropped to 248, 6 percent less than it had been forty-four years before. The picture for African-American women is even more discouraging. Initially, the government kept no records of breast cancer in black women. In 1973, the first year that such records were compiled, the death rate from breast cancer for black women was 263 for every 10,000. By 1995, it had soared to 319.

Many scientists believed those statistics could improve only with profound new insights into the nature of cancer itself. For almost a century, scientists have been raising research funds by promising that such breakthroughs were imminent. In 1898, Dr. Roswell Park, a surgeon in Buffalo, persuaded the New York State legislature to create the Institute for the Study of Malignant Disease by declaring that "the cure is just around the corner." The state built the institute, which was named after Roswell Park following his death. But the reality was that no one understood the fundamental biology of cancer—a word that covers approximately 110 distinct ailments.

The National Cancer Act, signed by Richard Nixon on December 23, 1971, amounted to a leap of faith based on exaggerated claims worthy of Roswell Park and on the perennial belief that the government can solve any problem by simply throwing money at it. The War on Cancer, as it was called, brought unheard-of sums of money to the field. Between 1971 and 1979, the budget of the National Cancer Institute climbed from $230 million to $940 million. Grant money did flow to cancer research, so much so that scientists seeking funding for other areas of basic research, like the fundamentals of the chemical reactions in cells, often justified their applications by fabricating some hypothetical application of their research to cancer. But in 1971, money was hardly the only obstacle standing in the way of a cure. Cancer research remained a scientific backwater where no one seemed to be making any headway. Most distinguished scientists regarded cancer research as a bastion of mediocrity where less talented scientists followed the money to perform meaningless experiments. Robert Weinberg, a pioneer in cancer research, recalls a senior colleague admonishing him "never, ever, under any circumstance, to confuse cancer research with science."

Cancer, the uncontrollable multiplication of cells, has existed from the moment single-celled organisms joined together to form multicelled plants and animals. Cancers have been found on dinosaur bones and on Egyptian mummies. Growing and dividing is the most basic function of individual cells. It is the impulse by which life has survived and evolved for billions of years. Every cell in our bodies carries this evolutionary force. But when cells band together to form a higher organism, they must answer to a more advanced impulse. Strict controls govern the proliferation of the body's individual cells. If the body's control mechanisms fail and individual cells reproduce beyond the limits of the system, cancer is the result.

What causes the deadly failure of control? Soon after the turn of the century researchers knew that radiation, chemicals, and viruses could trigger cancer. But this knowledge still failed to provide a satisfactory description of the actual change that is cancer itself.

With James Watson and Francis Crick's landmark discovery of the structure of DNA in 1953, alterations in genes, the units of heredity spelled out in the DNA molecule, became obvious candidates for cancer's cause. Watson and Crick's double helix offered nothing less that the master blueprint for all of life. It followed that the double helix also held the secret of cancer.

For centuries, biologists had theorized about the nature and function of genes, which are passed on from generation to generation and determine myriad characteristics, from physical traits to psychological dispositions. But until the Watson and Crick discovery, no one knew exactly what a gene was made of.

Suddenly, it was clear. The DNA molecule is made up of a string of millions of pairs of units, called nucleotides, that contain one of only four bases—adenine, cytosine, thymine, and guanine—that spell the genetic code. A single gene is a string of the ACTG alphabet that carries the instructions for the cell to make a particular protein. The proteins in turn usually provide one of two essential components: the cell's structural scaffolding or the enzymes that guide biochemical reactions—the central engine for the entire organism. So the genes contained in every cell encode information that determines not only how the individual cells look and behave but also how the entire organism looks and behaves. By establishing what proteins a cell produces, the genes on the DNA helix direct the formation of all life, from blades of grass to the human brain. Wouldn't abnormal changes to this master blueprint be responsible for cancer? This sounded plausible, especially since X rays and many of the chemicals that cause cancer also bring mutations to DNA. According to Robert Weinberg, many scientists believed that with the discovery of the DNA structure, "answers to the cancer problem would be all there, waiting to be discovered." But no one could prove a connection between genes and cancer until the mid-1970s, when new technologies for manipulating and understanding genes led to a revolution in the understanding of the disease.

Two researchers at the University of California, San Francisco, carried out the critical experiment that showed definitively that the roots of cancer lay in the genes of cells. Michael Bishop, a virologist, and his postdoctoral fellow, Harold Varmus, who went on to head the National Institutes of Health, were studying a chicken virus first discovered in 1911.

Viruses are the smallest bits of life—often called tiny packets of trouble. They never divide as cellular organisms, including bacteria, do. While bacteria and cells in higher creatures carry tens of thousands of genes, viruses make do with much less—often fewer than a dozen genes. Viruses survive from generation to generation because the viral genes carry the program for a commando raid. Usually when a virus infects a cell, its genes take over the control of a cell's machinery and transform the cell into a virus-making factory that eventually explodes, spewing out thousands of new viruses. But occasionally a virus employs a different strategy. It does not kill the cell but transforms it into a cancer cell. Other scientists had determined that only one gene in the cancer-causing chicken virus was responsible for the malignant transformation. What was this gene? What was this single unit of information that could cause cancer?

Initially, Bishop and Varmus—along with everyone else—thought that it was a viral gene. But certain viruses have a curious ability to act as gene kidnappers. Viruses occasionally capture a gene from a cell of the organism they invade and carry that gene as a passenger alongside its own set of genes. Bishop and Varmus found that the crucial cancer-causing gene was one of these accidental passengers carried by the virus. The Bishop and Varmus lab then determined that the gene dwells peacefully in chicken cells, where it performs some normal, harmless function. But in the virus, the same gene exists in a slightly mutated form.

The only conclusion—and it was a monumental one—was that within the normal chicken cell is a gene that, at least under some conditions, has the potential to cause cancer. In this case, a virus triggers the gene's potential to cause cancer. But soon experiments would show that other factors could coax the gene to cause cancer. It turns out that the switch that transforms a cell from normal to cancerous is a class of genes given the name oncogenes. The potentially cancer-causing genes, called proto-oncogenes in their normal state, perform functions critical to normal cellular behavior. But when these normal genes mutate to become oncogenes, they cause the cell to grow out of control into a potentially life-threatening mass.

This discovery of oncogenes brought mind-boggling implications: cancer might be triggered by some outside agent, such as radiation or chemicals, that might damage the gene, but the critical change actually takes place within the cell. Occasionally a human or other animal inherits an oncogene in the mutated form that gives rise to cancer. But far more often the gene mutates in the cell of the adult. Thus all cancer is genetic even if it is not usually inherited. In fact, all the cells of the body carry their own potential to become cancerous. With this first discovery came the rudiments of an accurate, detailed description of cancer. Only by understanding the foe could scientists even hope to devise significantly better ways of attacking it.

The Bishop-Varmus discovery set off a frenzy of research to find out exactly how oncogenes carry out their insidious cellular conversion. Before long, researchers identified just a handful of genes that appeared to cause a wide variety of cancers. Soon words like *src, myb, ras,* and *erb* permeated the lexicon of cancer researchers (by convention, cancer researchers usually give oncogenes three-letter names). One gene could somehow spark lung, colon, pancreatic, and dozens of other cancers. Amazingly, the particular genes whose mutations could lead to cancer in humans appeared throughout the animal kingdom. The same gene could be found in mice, people, ducks, even lowly yeast cells. These genes, which when altered could make normal cells multiply out of control, have persisted for hundreds of millions of years. Clearly, they survived intact because they performed some crucial function in the cells that evolution could not afford to discard. They also sowed the seeds of cancer and offered the tantalizing possibility of curing it.

At the time that Anne McNamara's cancer struck, Robert Weinberg, a thirty-one-year-old assistant professor at the Massachusetts Institute of Technology, led the pack of scientists chasing oncogenes. Loquacious and erudite, Weinberg is physically unprepossessing. Five foot six, he sports a bushy black mustache and combs his hair horizontally across the top of his balding head. He is that rare scientist able to communicate the significance of scientific achievements, his own or others', with great clarity, insight, and humor. Weinberg is always quick to point out that others in his lab did the actual work. "They feared my presence at the lab bench; I screwed everything up," he confesses.

Despite the professed deference Weinberg made huge contributions to basic research on cancer. He jumped into oncogene research as it was yielding its profound insights into the basic underpinnings of cancer. Among his earliest achievements was establishing that oncogenes themselves, not viruses, cause cancer. No one can say for certain what motivates the elders of the Karolinska Institute in Stockholm, but had Weinberg paid a bit more attention to a gene named neu, later Her-2/neu, he might have snared the great brass ring called the Nobel Prize.

The big challenge in 1979 for Weinberg and the tiny band of top scientists with whom he competed was to clone a pure sample of the DNA stretch that makes up an oncogene. By the late 1970s, the science of cloning was just giving birth to the biotechnology industry and allowing researchers to study genes in detail for the first time; though by today's standards, the early technology was primitive and the process very painstaking.

That year, while Anne McNamara was recovering from her surgery, a postdoctoral fellow in Weinberg's lab discovered neu.

Lakshmi Charon Padhy, a young researcher from Bombay, extracted DNA from neurological tumors in rats and injected it into normal mouse cells, which then turned cancerous. Padhy then discovered that sometimes these cancerous mouse cells trigger an immune response in the mice because of a particular rat protein now on the surface of the mouse cells, a product of one of the genes from the rat tumors. Weinberg dubbed the gene that produced the cancerous cells "neu" because it first appeared in tumors of the neurological system.

After naming neu, Weinberg more or less forgot about it. Over the years, he worked with it from time to time, but it never held a high priority. Other targets appeared more worthwhile. But as Weinberg would learn later, the neu protein was precisely the agent that the oncogene used to transform a normal cell into a cancer cell. If Weinberg had cloned neu, he would have had in hand the very protein the oncogene uses to make a cell cancerous. But Weinberg missed the opportunity and instead spent a frustrating two years trying to clone another oncogene called ras; it was produced in the neurological tumors Padhy and Weinberg were working with, but Weinberg went looking for it elsewhere.

"I can flagellate myself," Weinberg says now. "If I'd been more studious and more focused and not as monomaniacal about the ideas that I had at the time, I would have made that connection." Weinberg could have carried out the key experiment years ahead of his competitors. "It would have been an overnight experiment. We just didn't do it," he admits, adding, "That's life. I can't complain or be embittered. It's not as if I didn't have my share of good luck."

In the years to follow, achievements were such that, despite the missed opportunity of neu, Weinberg heard from friends that he would share a Nobel Prize with Bishop and Varmus. "Lots of people said to me, 'You're next, Bob.' " But when Bishop and Varmus got the award in 1989, there was no third winner. Weinberg, who won every significant honor in science save the big one, tries to remain philosophical. "How much do you need to make you happy?" he asks. "And in fifty years, who will care who won the Nobel Prize?"

No matter who got the credit, the discovery of oncogenes and the growing understanding of how they work revolutionized cancer research by providing the first understanding of the fundamental biology of the disease. A "magic bullet" therapy that would attack the disease at its root and halt its growth without inflicting any damage to healthy tissue had long been a dream in cancer treatment. But science needed a target. Now, finally, it had one. Researchers knew what they were looking for; they knew where to train their sights. In the late '70s and early '80s, scientists found dozens of oncogenes, along with a related class of genes called tumor suppressors that can also give rise to cancer. The neu oncogene, once bypassed by Weinberg, would play a key part in the struggle to bring the new genetic understanding of cancer out of the laboratory and to the patient's bedside.

CHAPTER 2

A Limited Arsenal

With her surgery behind her, Anne McNamara's life was blessedly uneventful. But in 1982, four years after her initial diagnosis, McNamara found a lump along her rib cage near the edge of her mastectomy scar. A few weeks later, at her next checkup, her surgeon wasn't initially concerned; it was probably just scar tissue. But a biopsy a week later revealed that it was malignant.

The McNamaras' growing sense of well-being was shattered. "I was pretty shaken," McNamara says. She should have been. Her luck had just taken the dramatic downturn that breast-cancer patients fear most. Her cancer was no longer a distant bad memory. It had reappeared as a real and present threat to her life. With its return, the disease assumes a new status, becoming what doctors euphemistically term "treatable but not curable." The battle may drag on for years, but the cancer almost always wins.

McNamara knew this, and she began planning for her funeral. She was not being melodramatic; she was being realistic.

"I thought about it, yeah. I thought of a friend who had died, and I went to her funeral," she says. "It was a memorial service. It was very nice and I liked it, and I thought I'd better think about what I want. And set something down, so that poor Jeff won't have to. I like a memorial service. I don't like funerals. I don't like calling hours. I don't like viewings. I don't like any of that. So, I was thinking, What hymns do I want? Very morbid. I couldn't talk to Jeff— he'd get very upset when I started talking about it, couldn't deal with it. He thinks it's wrong to dwell on things. But I was. I was thinking about it now. How am I going to know what hymns I like?

"I said, 'Well, this is it, and I've entered that club, and the end is in sight.' That's a very frightening thing to face. Before, I had never really thought that I would die. Then I did." This time, McNamara knew that chemotherapy was unavoidable.

McNamara's oncologist prescribed the standard combination of drugs: Cytoxan, methotrexate, and fluorouracil (also known as 5-FU), a cocktail commonly referred to as CMF. Every two to three weeks over the next six months, she drove to her local hospital for an infusion. McNamara knew how physically devastating chemotherapy can be, so she felt fortunate that the worst side effects she suffered were relatively mild nausea and thinning hair. But there was one side effect that she hadn't expected: she stopped menstruating.

After the chemotherapy ended, her periods returned, but only temporarily. What she did not know was that CMF often renders women infertile, especially women close to forty, and can induce premature menopause. By the time she turned forty, McNamara had stopped menstruating altogether. Although she had already made the decision not to get pregnant again, she is still angry. "I just think it never occurred to them that it was important," she says. It is precisely that kind of indifference toward the concerns of female patients that sparked the women's health movement of the 1970s. One measure of effectiveness of the movement is that now many patients are better briefed about treatments and their potential side effects so that they can make informed choices. McNamara acknowledges that once her cancer recurred, she really had no choice. Chemotherapy—even with its possible negative consequences—was the best hope for long-term survival that modern medicine could offer her.

Though McNamara's treatment options were narrow, they were better than they had been for women thirty, twenty, or even ten years earlier. Yet improvements in breast-cancer treatment have been agonizingly slow to appear, and nothing has approached the universal goal of a cure. Surgery, radiation, chemotherapy, and hormone treatment all boost both life expectancy and quality of life for breast-cancer survivors. But the stagnant death rates starkly demonstrate how little genuine progress has occurred and how great the need is for new treatments.

Surgery has been part of the arsenal for centuries. Doctors have long recognized that the most effective way to deal with cancer is to find it early and remove it. If it spreads internally, the outlook is grim. But before the use of anesthesia and sterile procedures became commonplace in the late nineteenth century, surgery often did more harm than good. Terrifying first-person accounts tell of women who underwent mastectomies performed by surgeons using nothing but knives heated until they glowed to cauterize the wounds.

Radiation therapy appeared as an option soon after the discovery of X rays, then radium in the 1890s. A tinkerer in Chicago named Emil Grubbe claimed to be the first person to treat breast cancer with radiation. Details of Wilhelm Röntgen's discovery of X rays in 1895 appeared in Chicago newspapers, and Grubbe, like many amateur scientists around the world, put together the proper arrangement of cathode-ray tubes to produce his own X-ray device. It did not take long for Grubbe to learn that the new rays could be dangerous. He severely burned his hands while fiddling with his machine. When he sought treatment at Hahneman Medical College, he inadvertently gave his doctors an idea. Relying on the ancient homeopathic belief that if a lot of something is harmful, a little should be helpful, they sent Mrs. Rose Lee, a fifty-five-year old with recurrent breast cancer, to Grubbe, and he claimed the X rays shrank her tumor. No reliable records exist of Mrs. Lee's recovery, but doctors around the world soon learned that radiation can treat cancer, although the danger of harming normal tissue is ever present.

Through the middle part of the twentieth century both radiation and surgery steadily improved. According to the American Cancer Society, the number of cancer patients living five years after their diagnosis jumped from one in five in 1930 to one in three in 1960— the greatest advance in cancer survival rates ever witnessed. But there the improvement stalled. Antibiotics, the polio vaccine, and better medications for all sorts of other conditions transformed most doctors, in the eyes of the public, into miracle workers who could conquer any malady. But all too often doctors had little to offer cancer patients beyond comfort and compassion. Seeking their own magic, cancer specialists turned to chemotherapy.

A tragedy off the Italian coast in 1943 offered a major clue for future cancer care. Merchant vessels and warships of the Allied forces were gathered in Bari Harbor one day when German bombers launched a surprise attack, raining fire on the ships below. One of the vessels that took a direct hit was the U.S.S. *John Harvey,* a cargo ship loaded with one hundred tons of mustard gas. Even though an international treaty outlawed the use of chemical weapons after World War I, President Franklin Roosevelt did not trust the enemy to abide by the agreement, so he insisted that the U.S. forces be equipped with them. As the *John Harvey* sank, its slimy contents oozed into the bay and mixed with burning oil. Sailors, fishermen, and other civilians from damaged ships were left flailing in the contaminated water. Within hours, military field hospitals were overflowing with the injured, many of them in agony with burning eyes, enormous blisters, and lungs filled with blood—all symptoms of mustard gas contact. Eighty-three sailors and one thousand others died.

The tragedy yielded a serendipitous result. Autopsies revealed something of tremendous importance to cancer researchers: the gas had primarily attacked the white blood cells, which divide more rapidly than most other cells in the body. Since frequent cell division is the hallmark of most cancer cells, this discovery suggested that a form of nitrogen mustard, one of the main ingredients of mustard gas, in lower doses might be used to kill rapidly dividing cancer cells.

The idea held special appeal for one of the most influential figures in cancer treatment at the time, Cornelius "Dusty" Rhoads. During the war, Rhoads was persuaded to take a leave from his prestigious post as head of New York City's Memorial Hospital (now Memorial Sloan Kettering Cancer Center) to run the military's chemical-warfare service. At the Edgewood Arsenal in Maryland, he supervised the long-secret and now-infamous tests in which thousands of American troops were intentionally exposed to mustard and other poisonous gases. Those experiments corroborated the evidence from the Bari autopsies. Even before the war ended, Rhoads and others began to experiment with mustard-gas derivatives as cancer treatments while searching for other systemic poisons that kill rapidly dividing cells. The pace of those experiments picked up when the war ended.

A young doctor, Sidney Farber, decided to try mixtures of various cell poisons to treat leukemia and the other cancers, mostly of the blood, that strike children. Initial attempts were heartbreaking. Often the poisons killed the children faster than they did the cancer, and even if the treatment wasn't lethal, the side effects of the chemotherapy brought intense misery. The problem was that the drugs attacked all the cells that divided rapidly, not just cancerous ones. Thus, while chemotherapy kills cancer cells, it also kills hair-follicle cells (causing rapid hair loss), cells lining the gut (bringing on intense nausea), and bone-marrow cells (leading to profound weakness and life-threatening anemia). But Farber persisted and refined his therapy, and soon he was effecting remissions and even cures in children who had faced an almost certain death.

Those successes sparked great hope that chemotherapy would treat not only leukemia but also all forms of cancer. In 1953, Dusty Rhodes, back in charge of Memorial Hospital, told a *New York Times* reporter, "Inevitably, as I see it, we can look forward to something like a penicillin for cancer, and I hope, within the next decade." But success against the major killer cancers fell far short of Rhode's hopes.

Breast cancer seemed to respond better than many cancers to chemotherapy. The three drugs Anne McNamara received in 1982 were hardly new. Methotrexate won FDA approval in 1953, cyclophosphamide (or Cytoxan) was approved in 1959, and fluorouracil (or 5-FU), in 1962. In 1974 the FDA approved the first drug specifically for breast cancer: Adriamycin (also known as doxorubicin). Like the three earlier drugs it interferes with DNA synthesis but its more powerful cancer-killing abilities are matched by its more distressing and dangerous side effects. In addition to nausea, hair loss, and bone-marrow destruction, Adriamycin can erode the heart muscle, leading to irreversible damage, with symptoms ranging from shortness of breath to death.

It was not until 1994 that the FDA approved a drug for breast cancer with a substantially different method of attack. Taxol, first approved as a treatment for ovarian cancer in 1992, received enormous media attention because it initially came from just one source, the bark of the scarce Pacific yew tree. It became a lightning rod for environmentalists, and news accounts often portrayed the Taxol issue as a choice between saving trees or cancer patients. But soon chemists found less-threatened sources for Taxol and developed a synthetic version, called Taxotere. Taxol and Taxotere kill cancer cells by interfering with crucial bodies outside the cell nucleus called microtubules, which function as the cell's skeleton. Taxol can be more effective than the other drugs, but it is no miracle cure. These five drugs—Taxol, Adriamycin, 5-FU, Cytoxan, and methotrexate—remain the primary drugs for the treatment of breast cancer to this day.

Large studies proved that used alone and in combination these drugs often shrank tumors—at least temporarily. Other trials proved that adjuvant chemotherapy can shift the odds against breast cancer recurring. But if the cancer reappeared, the prognosis remained bleak. The outlook seemed to differ little from the first century A.D. when the great Roman medical chronicler Celsus wrote, "Only the beginning of a cancer admits of a cure."

When her cancer returned in 1982, McNamara's doctor prescribed a round of CMF, and he also put her on a yearlong course of tamoxifen, an estrogen blocker. On this drug, she suffered nothing worse than such mild menopausal symptoms as hot flashes. The doctor's strategy was to attack the disease on two fronts: attempt to kill the rogue cells with chemotherapy and, given that McNamara's tumor was shown to feed on estrogen, starve the disease by denying it the hormone it needed to grow and spread.

Hormone treatment marked the first step away from the familiar triad of surgery, radiation, and chemotherapy—the "slash, burn, and poison" so memorably labeled by Susan Love. Its roots go back a century. In 1896 Sir George Beatson described a new method for treating advanced breast cancer in young women—castration, or surgical removal of the ovaries. An accomplished surgeon, Beatson knew that farmers in his native Scotland had understood for generations that they could boost a cow's milk production by removing her ovaries. He guessed that removing a woman's ovaries would affect her breast tissue and, in the case of breast cancer, perhaps slow tumor growth. After practicing on rabbits, he tried the procedure in three young women. In all the cases the tumors shrank and the women's conditions seemed to improve, at least temporarily. But, as so often happens with early treatments of advanced cancer, the disease returned and killed the patients. Beatson concluded his report in *The Lancet,* an important British medical journal, with a disclaimer that would accompany almost every discovery in cancer treatment for the next one hundred years: "I know that I have had nothing in the way of great results, but it must be remembered that I have worked with the most unpromising cases."

Beatson's results remained puzzling until the discovery of estrogen-receptor (ER) molecules in certain cells that receive the signal carried by the female hormone estrogen. When the estrogen attaches to the receptor, it tells the cell to carry out a task, such as ovulation, menstruation, pregnancy, or lactation. Estrogen's activity was one of the first examples of the critical process called cell signaling, the means by which all cells in the body receive messages, including orders to grow and divide. Some, but not all, breast-cancer cells carry estrogen receptors. When a breast cancer cell carries a receptor, the grow-and-divide message from the estrogen molecule can be crucial for its proliferation. About 40 percent of breast cancers in premenopausal women (including Anne McNamara) and 60 percent in postmenopausal women are ER positive. Tumors that are ER positive tend to be less life threatening than those that are ER negative, precisely because they respond to estrogen therapy.

Blocking the estrogen receptor emerged as an obvious target for drug development. Eventually, a failed contraceptive produced by ICI, the British chemical giant (now known as Zeneca Pharmaceuticals), and developed by V. Craig Jordan, now at Northwestern University, accomplished the task. Tamoxifen won approval from the Committee on the Safety of Drugs in the United Kingdom in 1973 and from the U.S. Food and Drug Administration in 1977 as a treatment for advanced breast cancer. Almost immediately, however, doctors began using it to treat the disease in earlier stages. In 1998, the standard of care dictates that most women with

ER-positive tumors get tamoxifen as preventive therapy soon after surgery, whether they get chemotherapy or not.

Soon after doctors began to use tamoxifen to treat women with breast cancer, they noticed that women taking the drug developed fewer new cancers in the nonaffected breast than women who did not take the drug. Dr. Bernard Fisher, a pioneering surgeon who ran clinical trials proving the benefits of adjuvant chemotherapy and of lumpectomy in place of mastectomy, saw that observation as an opportunity to try to prevent breast cancer entirely. He applied for funds for a massive clinical trial. It enrolled more than thirteen thousand women considered to be at high risk for breast cancer because they had a family history of the disease, were age sixty or older, or fit one of several other criteria. Half received a placebo, a dummy pill. The other half received tamoxifen. In April 1998 the results revealed that women taking tamoxifen were 45 percent less likely to develop breast cancer. Because of the drug's side effects, including an increased risk of blood clots and uterine cancer, healthy women did not stampede to get it. A second estrogen blocker, called raloxifene, soon appeared to be a possibly better bet. Two-year results presented in May 1998 revealed that it reduced breast cancer by 58 percent without the side effects. Many doctors believed that a new era of breast-cancer prevention was beginning, but whatever the possibility of prevention, the concept came too late for women like Anne McNamara stricken with the disease.

McNamara faced a second recurrence of the disease in 1987. During a regular checkup, her oncologist found a swollen lymph node just above her collarbone. He was not alarmed and recommended waiting a month to see if the swelling would go down. McNamara knew the swelling wasn't a fluke. Once again her instincts led her to challenge her doctor's recommendation. She refused to wait a month. "I hated the waiting and the not knowing," she says.

Two weeks later, she went in for a biopsy, and sure enough the node was malignant. Her doctor prescribed six weeks of radiation to eradicate any remaining cancer cells. The treatments themselves last just a few minutes and can bring on nausea, muscle aches, swelling, and skin redness. McNamara was most uncomfortable when she had to lie on her side with her left arm extended way back over her head; that position stretched her mastectomy scar. The therapy ended, and McNamara, as she had after her mastectomy and after the first recurrence, went back to her life with her husband and son, who was now ten, and hoped for the best, even as her hope was faltering.

Anne's husband, Jeff, acknowledges that since his wife's cancer first emerged, life changed in a number of ways. "It affects priorities," he says, in his down-to-earth fashion. "I'm a more generous nature. I'm not blowing my own horn. I've made every effort to do things with Annie and with our son just because next year she may not be around. For example, travel. We've done a lot of traveling. Fortunately, we've been able to and have done some neat things. The first ten years, I did that, and encouraged her. You know, she would hang back, but I would say, 'Come on, come on, come on.' "

Anne McNamara's ongoing battle against recurrent disease represented the best medicine had to offer women with breast cancer at the time: surgery, radiation, chemotherapy, and hormone treatment. All of these could stall some of breast cancer's momentum, but each took a heavy toll, and none offered the solid promise of a cure. Everyone wanted better treatments. And almost every scientist and researcher had great expectations, certain that a whole new way of treating breast cancer would come from the study of oncogenes and the ever-deepening understanding of the genetic basis of cancer.

CHAPTER 3

A New Way
of Doing Science

As often happens in science, the research that led to an important innovation in cancer treatment began not with hundreds of scientists working toward a stated goal but with a lone researcher who happened onto the trail by accident. In the case of the first gene-based cancer treatment, that person worked not for the government, academia, or a giant pharmaceutical company, the three traditional loci of medical research, but for that infant phenomenon of the late 1970s and early '80s: the biotechnology industry.

Axel Ullrich did not set out to break one of cancer's secret codes. He was universally recognized as a master cloner, a wizard at isolating the specific stretches of DNA that comprise genes. He likes to boast of his scientific exploits, great insights that he says were ahead of their time. "That was sort of the story of my life," he says without a trace of irony. "That I had all these ideas that people were not quite ready for, and yet then I leave, and then they reinvent the idea." Ullrich possesses the rugged good looks and swagger of an American cowboy. When he talks, he sounds like Henry Kissinger.

Educated through the doctorate level in his native Germany, he won a postdoctoral fellowship in the Biochemistry Department of the University of California at San Francisco. There could be no more exciting place for a young biologist to be. There he witnessed the birth of biotechnology and made his own contributions to it. When Ullrich arrived at UCSF in 1975, Bishop and Varmus were down the hall working on their chicken oncogene, and their colleague Herb Boyer was helping develop the technology of gene splicing, the critical tool of genetic engineering. Boyer would soon cofound Genentech, one of the first companies to exploit the new techniques of genetic engineering.

One of Ullrich's achievements at UCSF was to isolate the gene that produces insulin in rats and transfer it into bacteria, thereby transforming them into microscopic insulin factories. This was the first time anyone had induced bacteria to produce a mammalian protein, the premier demonstration of the very technique that would form the backbone of the biotechnology industry. But that triumph turned sour at a press conference called to announce this discovery. Ullrich's supervisor, who had been on sabbatical when most of the work was done and had discouraged him from pursuing his hypothesis, swooped in to stand before the cameras and take all the credit. Ullrich was left looking like a bit player. He determined never to let himself be burned like that again.

Along with several of his colleagues at UCSF, Ullrich eventually moved to South San Francisco to work at the newly founded Genentech, although he resisted at first. In 1977, Robert Swanson, the twenty-seven-year-old venture capitalist who had cofounded the company with Boyer, nearly succeeded in luring Ullrich away from the university. At the last minute Ullrich told him that he feared he might never be allowed to return to academic research if he joined what was then a suspect enterprise. Swanson tore up his contract. Six months later, Ullrich finally made the jump. He acknowledges that the six-month delay cost him $10 million in Genentech stock and laughs at the thought, displaying a gambler's nonchalance about fortunes lost and won on the frontier of biotechnology. He can afford to laugh: over the years, he has made back that loss and much more.

But more alluring than the money, according to Ullrich, was Swanson's willingness to allow the top scientists to carry out their own research virtually unfettered by the traditional standards of the drug industry and other profit-making corporations that sponsor research. The new Genentech scientists would have almost the same freedom as those in universities to pursue whatever ideas they chose. Corporate scientists, often working in secret, carried out applied science—directed toward the goal of creating a product. Says Ullrich, "We just convinced Bob Swanson that he had to allow us to publish and publish fast and be in contact with the academic scientific community. And that became the basis of this completely new way of doing science," an approach that would prove productive both for basic science and for drug discovery.

Genentech was not the first biotechnology company—Cetus, across the bay in Berkeley, had opened its doors in 1971. Nor was it the most successful—Amgen in southern California earned greater profits. But on October 14, 1980, Genentech's initial public stock offering soared from thirty-five dollars per share to eighty-nine dollars in the first twenty minutes of trading and closed that day at just about seventy dollars. This unprecedented performance instantly made Genentech the avatar of a fledgling industry synonymous with great risk and great reward. Wall Street had clearly discovered biotechnology.

The very essence of biotechnology was the arrangement Ullrich and the other young scientists won from Swanson. The early biotechnologists believed they would carry out research of the highest quality and then turn the results into new drugs with a swiftness that the staid pharmaceutical industry could not match. In the years before the industry emerged, the pharmaceutical giants ("big pharma," in the lexicon of biotechnology) rarely carried out experiments without having a clear goal. For the most part, they left pure research to the scientists at university and government labs. Drug-company scientists concentrated on the often boring and repetitious steps necessary either to find a drug at random or to convert someone else's basic research discovery into a useful medicine. Genentech's bravado was rooted in the then novel idea that the same scientists could carry out top-notch basic research, be instantly aware of its potential for drug development, and help bring it to market. In time, researchers would realize some limitations to this approach. But in the early days, they saw none.

Ullrich's first foray into cancer research involved a critically important chemical called epidermal growth factor. As the name implies, EGF helps control the growth of the epidermis, or skin. Like estrogen, EGF belongs to a class of chemicals, called growth factors, that carry orders that regulate not just growth but every body function, from food digestion and blood pressure to sleeping and breathing. (A chemical that carries such signals through the entire body is called a hormone. But not all growth factors travel through the body; EGF, for example, only goes from one cell to the next.) Because of their important role in so many processes, these chemicals were of great interest to scientists at Genentech and elsewhere who believed they held the key to understanding many fundamentals of physiology. With that understanding, these scientists could develop drugs to combat many kinds of ailments.

While the chemical orders move through the body, they do not deliver their messages to every cell. Like the handful of children in a classroom who raise their hands in response to an assignment, only a few cells are inclined to get the message. In fact, the only cells that understand the chemical's message are those that carry a receptor, a specific antenna-like protein on the cell's surface. EGF's orders are always the same—to grow and divide—and to deliver them, it attaches to the EGF receptor on a cell's surface.

Just before Christmas in 1983, Ullrich got a phone call from Mike Waterfield, a top protein chemist in London. Waterfield believed he might have the first evidence of what an oncogene actually does to cause cancer. Many scientists had postulated but not yet proved that oncogenes are related to chemicals like EGF, which control growth. But Waterfield had the proof. He told Ullrich he had purified the protein that acts as the EGF receptor. Based on the structure of the protein, Waterfield had an inkling that the EGF receptor was not just related to the protein product of an oncogene called erb-b, which causes a blood cancer in chickens, but was identical to it. Waterfield needed Ullrich to join him in London to clone the gene for the human EGF receptor by working backward from the structure of the protein.

With the gene in hand, Waterfield, Ullrich, and an Israeli protein expert named Joseph Schlessinger were able to offer the first experimental proof of the extraordinarily important theory that growth factors are related to cancer. They showed that the oncogene called erb-b is indeed a mutated form of the gene that programs the receptor for EGF. In early 1984, the three men published their landmark findings in the prestigious journal *Nature*.

Their conclusion was a milestone in cancer research because it drew a critical connection between what had been two separate areas of biology—the study of cell-growth signals and the study of cancer—and for the first time explained how an oncogene works. When functioning normally, the gene regulates the delicate ballet of cell growth and division. When mutated, it brings on unrestrained growth—cancer. Almost all oncogenes turn out to be mutated forms of the genes that regulate cell growth and division. In just a decade and a half, that discovery became so widely accepted that it was soon taught in high-school biology classes.

Back from London, Ullrich began searching human DNA for genes similar to the EGF-receptor gene. The first one he found he named Her-2 for *h*uman-*e*pidermal-growth-factor *r*eceptor-2 (the gene he had cloned for Waterfield would have been Her-1, but it had another name before Waterfield ever connected it to cancer).

With existing cloning technology, Ullrich could determine what protein the gene produced. It was the same one that had appeared on the cancerous mouse cells in Robert Weinberg's lab in 1979 and had led to the discovery of the neu oncogene. From a completely different direction, Ullrich had rediscovered neu. Now he had both the gene and the protein in hand. What would have been an unprecedented accomplishment five years earlier was now but one more signpost on the long road to discovering how oncogenes work. When Ullrich presented the data on Her-2 in late 1984, Weinberg heard about it and immediately understood what he had missed. It was a poignant realization. "For want of a nail," he says philosophically, "a small kingdom fell." The gene is now commonly known as Her-2/neu in deference to both scientists' work.*

Cloning growth factors and their target receptors had been Ullrich's and Genentech's specialty. Genentech's first major accomplishment was cloning human insulin, a growth factor produced in the pancreas that tells the liver and muscles to absorb glucose. Genentech licensed that technology to Eli Lilly. The first treatment Genentech itself produced was human growth hormone, which stimulates growth throughout the body. The company eventually sold it as a drug designed to help prevent dwarfism in children.

Ullrich had amassed his own collection of growth factor and receptor genes; now he wanted to find out if any of them play a role in cancer's onset or progression.

The door to the next discovery opened at Denver's Stapleton International Airport in the spring of 1986. Ullrich had ducked out of a disappointing scientific conference and was heading home early. While waiting for his flight, he met another conference at-

---

* To make matters more confusing, the gene is also called erb-b-2 because of its origin in the erb-b oncogene. Two other groups discovered the gene at about the same time.

tendee who evidently had the same reaction. The man was Dennis Slamon. The two men had seen each other at the meeting but had never met. Over drinks they talked of their research and decided that a collaboration someday could prove beneficial, but their departure times arrived before they got close to any details.

Slamon is a practicing oncologist with a doctorate in cell biology and a savage will to attain a single goal—a treatment for cancer so superior that it will earn him a place in the textbooks. Even at rest, he's never still, usually twitching his graying mustache—a sign to those who know him that his mind has ambled ahead to his next meeting, conference, or patient visit. Despite a schedule already overflowing, he seems unable to resist additional responsibilities. In an attempt to meet his obligations, he pares away the day's nonessential activities, like returning phone calls. He admits that he seldom saw his children during the first decade of their lives. Conversation for him can be difficult, almost as if he regards it as an inconvenience. When he is forced to converse, he is all nervous energy, coiled to spring out of his seat.

It is only when he talks about the science of his work and its clinical applications that he finally seems to relax. At these moments, he is spirited, focused, even full of humor, his devotion to the cause animating his expressive eyes and gestures. Research is, after all, his passion—his ongoing passage out of the destitution of his childhood.

Slamon is muscular and tall, looking as though he easily could have followed family tradition and gone to work in the coal mines of Appalachia. In 1913, his grandfather, Ahmed, emigrated with his family from their Syrian village to West Virginia and Pennsylvania, where he searched for work digging coal. All three of his sons joined him in the mines. His youngest, Joseph, married an American and had three children. Joseph left the mines after he, his father, and his brother twice had to be dug out of cave-ins. "He wasn't going to go down anymore," Dennis recalls of his father with a trace of Appalachian twang still echoing in his speech. Joseph put the dangers of coal mining behind him and took a job driving a Coca-Cola truck. But he was in a terrible wreck that cost him a leg and two years in the hospital. Dennis was two at the time; his two older sisters were forced to find work to support the family.

Dennis's excellent high-school grades won him a scholarship to Washington and Jefferson, a small college in Washington, Pennsylvania. He was the first in his family to get a college education. In the summer between college and medical school, he met and married Donna Williamson, a tall, attractive woman who was working as a lifeguard at a local swimming pool. Slamon says he had always wanted to be a physician because of the enormous respect his family accorded the doctors who came to the house to tend to his injured father. From Washington and Jefferson, he won a full scholarship to the combination MD-PhD program at the University of Chicago.

Slamon entered the field of medical research at a time when the money from the War on Cancer was flowing freely into laboratories across the country. He did his graduate work under two leading molecular biologists, Winston Anderson and Werner Kirstein, who were studying cell growth and division and their possible relationship to cancer. After earning his dual degree in 1975, he remained at the University of Chicago for his internship and residency. The following year, Bishop and Varmus published their landmark paper on the discovery of the first oncogene. The field of oncology, which had been mired for so long in the backwaters of science, exploded with excitement, attracting a generation of very bright young men and women, including Dennis Slamon.

In 1979, when Slamon finished his residency, he chose from his many options a fellowship, a junior faculty position, in the Department of Hematology-Oncology at the University of California,

Los Angeles. (In academic hospitals, the oncology specialty grew out of the hematology departments because it achieved its initial successes with leukemias and other cancers of the blood. By the 1980s, many hospitals had established separate oncology departments.) Slamon divided his time between research and patient care. Like thousands of other scientists and research clinicians in the late 1970s, Slamon saw oncogenes as the brightest light yet to illuminate the darkness of cancer.

A faculty member at UCLA, Slamon always preferred the lab bench to the bedside. "The clinical aspects of oncology are not attractive," he says. "It's not fun to deal with patients who have potentially life-threatening diseases day in and day out." Slamon's patients describe him as caring and attentive, but his heart is really in the pursuit of a cure. To that end, he had what struck many as a bizarre hobby: he collected freshly excised human tumors—lung, liver, breast, colon, whatever he could get from surgeons and pathologists. Even he describes this pastime as ghoulish, but he believed that his collection held the secrets of cancer's origins.

Many specialists regarded Slamon's pursuit as a fool's errand. They believed that oncogenes could be found only in the neat lines of millions of identical cancer cells cultured in petri dishes. The difference between a normal cell and a cancer cell amounts to only a few tiny mutations among the cell's one hundred thousand genes. A tumor is far more than a knot of cancer cells; it is composed of many kinds of tissue, blood, and lymph. Finding an oncogene in a petri dish is difficult enough. Finding one in a tumor, the scientists reasoned, is close to impossible.

A few months after the airport meeting, Ullrich was at UCLA giving a seminar. Slamon took the opportunity to make a suggestion. He knew that Ullrich had genes for growth factors, the chemicals that carry grow-and-divide signals through the body. Slamon wanted to know which of these genes, if any, caused cancer. Slamon's own collection of cancer tissues seemed like a natural place to look for links between Ullrich's growth-factor genes and specific types of human cancer. Collaboration made sense. The two sealed a deal over a long dinner at a Thai restaurant in Santa Monica: Ullrich would send Slamon samples of DNA from his gene collection, and Slamon would try to match them to the DNA he had extracted from his tumor collection.

Ullrich did not inform Genentech of the experiments. He boasts that he flouted the corporate rules all the time. But while he did not seek permission from Genentech, he did protect the company's patent rights by disguising with code names the identities of the samples he sent to Slamon. Slamon put Wendy Levin, his undergraduate assistant (the usual graduate or postdoctoral student was beyond his financial reach), to work ferreting out matches between the oncogenes and the tumors. One of Ullrich's genes scored a match with certain breast and ovarian cancers. Slamon called Ullrich: "We got a hit." Ullrich then revealed that the gene was called Her-2/neu.

Slamon and Ullrich set out to find out how Her-2/neu was connected to cancerous growth in breast and ovarian cells. They discovered that this oncogene had not mutated like most others; usually, a mutation causes the gene to produce either a defective protein or no protein at all. With Her-2/neu, the affected cells produce the normal protein, but in abnormally high amounts. This is a phenomenon in molecular biology known as overexpression. Further studies showed that the Her-2/neu gene's protein appears on the cell surface as a receptor, similar to the EGF receptor. It, too, is an antenna that receives signals telling the cell to grow and divide. When the gene is mutated and overexpresses the protein, the cell is overloaded with signals that cause it to grow out of control—to become cancerous. A typical breast cell carries about 50,000 Her-2/neu receptors on its surface. When the gene is mutated the number jumps to between 1 and 1.5 million.

Reflecting on the experiment years later, Ullrich emphasizes that he and Slamon enjoyed "an amazing amount of luck." Ullrich tried to find other oncogenes using the same DNA-matching technology. He tried to match DNA from 150 suspected oncogenes with the DNA from tumor cells just the way Slamon had, and he did not get a single hit. "We haven't found anything. Her-2 is the only one that sticks out of the crowd." And Her-2 offered another bit of serendipity. The receptor protein protrudes from the cell surface, creating an accessible target for something therapeutic. Most other oncogene mutations disrupt the chemistry deep within the cell, causing changes that are much more difficult to get at.

Until the moment Axel Ullrich introduced Dennis Slamon to Her-2, the oncologist hadn't studied women's cancers specifically. In the clinic, he treated all forms of cancer, and in his lab he searched for oncogenes that might apply to any tumor type. But from then on, Her-2/neu would be the obsessive force in his professional life. Over the years, other researchers have ridiculed him for focusing on a single gene that few believed would ever yield a treatment. With the gene's connection to breast cancer established, he turned his attention to finding out what kinds of breast cancers are associated with Her-2/neu. His own collection of thirty breast-cancer tumors would be no help because he had no histories for them: he did not know how the women from whom they had been removed had responded to treatment. So Slamon turned to Bill McGuire, a legendary researcher in San Antonio who had spent years studying the hormones estrogen and progesterone and their effects on breast cancer. McGuire had a sizable collection of frozen tumors with detailed medical histories and assigned a young associate Gary Clark to work with Slamon.

Clark and Slamon designed an experiment in which Slamon measured each tumor's Her-2/neu status without knowing the patient's history. The results suggested that the cancers that overexpress Her-2 are deadlier, more apt to recur, and spread faster than other cancers. The discovery meant it would be easier to predict which cancers are most likely to recur—one of the greatest challenges in treating the disease. The most reliable tool for making such predictions had been, at best, imprecise: counting the number of cancerous lymph nodes before mastectomy. Slamon, along with Ullrich, McGuire, Clark, and Levin, were offering oncology a diagnostic tool far more reliable and more precise. They published their findings in the prestigious journal *Science* in January 1987. Printed under a full-page headline, the article trumpeted a major advance in the understanding and treatment of breast cancer.

Then the first in a long series of setbacks struck the Her-2 research.

Almost as soon as the journal reached its readers, researchers throughout the United States and the world began to grouse that they could not duplicate the experiment, a problem that instantly threw the article's claims into question. To maintain one's credibility as a researcher, it is not enough to stake a claim on a scientific discovery; others must be able to perform the same experiment with identical results. Perhaps the research community would have been less critical had Slamon been someone prominent. But he was an unknown, and the scientific world, like every other, has its hierarchy. Scientists tend to believe results more readily if they come from expected sources.

Not only was Slamon unknown, but in the 1980s, UCLA was viewed as a second-rate research institution, hardly in the same class as the molecular-biology powerhouses, such as the University of California, San Francisco, and MIT. To make matters worse, when Slamon first arrived at UCLA, he settled into the laboratory of Martin Cline, a researcher who had gained widespread notoriety in 1980 for traveling to Israel and Italy to conduct gene-therapy experiments that were then banned in the United States. Cline's experiments turned out to be unsuccessful, UCLA reprimanded him, and the National Institutes of Health rescinded much of his financial support. Slamon had absolutely nothing to do with those experiments, but such scandals—rare as they are—cast a wide net of suspicion.

Over the next two years, Slamon and Ullrich fought what seemed to be universal dismissal. First they set out to repeat their experiment successfully with many more breast tumors. Finding physicians willing to donate specimens proved difficult. Slamon remembers in particular that Larry Norton at Sloan Kettering evidenced no desire to assist with what he saw as a useless effort. Eventually they collected enough tumors to complete the experiment. Then they took their campaign a step further: they meticulously proved that the other laboratories that had failed to reproduce the experiment had foundered on contaminated chemicals, faulty techniques, and idiotic mistakes. The failed attempts to confirm the *Science* paper "were done by MDs, and not all MDs are good scientists and, especially technically, [are] not so experienced," explains Ullrich. "There was a lot of garbage." He and Slamon published a second paper in *Science* in May 1989. This time they proved the original results more forcefully. Still the scientific community, for the most part, wasn't interested in taking a second look. In research, as elsewhere, first impressions count. Even though their evidence had been solid all along, Slamon and Ullrich's work was tarnished by the initial skepticism.

Slamon remains philosophical about the situation. "Things like that build character," he says. "We all felt good about what we were doing, but we wasted two years because someone had not done careful science." The lost time was bad enough, but it turned out to be just the first in a string of frustrating delays in bringing an important new diagnostic tool and, eventually, a treatment to patients. Even science and medicine have their fads and fashions. Many academic physicians make decisions based not so much on a careful study of scientific literature as on the talk that accompanies the latest new and much-discussed discovery. Her-2/neu burned brightly in their minds for an instant but grew increasingly dim in the initial backwash of criticism. Even after Slamon had disproved his critics, it took his research years to recover from the blow.

Despite the rejection, Slamon, ever determined, continued to accumulate impressive results. At Genentech, a small group of researchers under Ullrich joined the effort, working on the basic science with an eye toward developing a drug. Using pure DNA copies of the Her-2/neu gene, they transformed normal cells growing in petri dishes into malignancies. Next, in what would be the crucial first step toward a treatment, they showed that they could shut off the gene and force the cancerous cells to become normal again. To accomplish this, Ullrich turned to Genentech's experienced Immunology Division and asked its researchers to produce monoclonal antibodies against the Her-2/neu protein. Antibodies are proteins that the body produces to combat bacterial and viral infection by latching on to a specific target, such as a molecule on the bacteria's surface. Millions of different antibodies defend the body against a vast array of invaders. A monoclonal antibody is a laboratory-manufactured solution containing millions of identical copies of a single antibody, all of which attack precisely the same target. Not wanting to work solely with Genentech, Slamon also obtained antibodies from other companies and university labs.

When Ullrich and Slamon added the monoclonal antibody to breast-cancer cells that overexpress Her-2/neu, the antibody shut down the Her-2/neu protein. Amazingly, the cancerous cells stopped growing and dividing. The antibody had no effect on other cells in the dish. When the researchers washed the antibody away, the cancerous growth returned. "It was fantastic," Slamon recalls. No one could doubt that Her-2/neu was an oncogene involved in particularly aggressive forms of breast cancer that resist treatment. The antibody's effect, like an on-off switch, suggested that the Her-2/neu gene could be the target of a revolutionary treatment, one that attacked the problem without bringing harm to healthy tissue. It was a stunning realization.

Meanwhile, out of the blue, Slamon got a call from a cancer researcher in Houston named Pepino Giovanella, who offered him a magnificent tool for further research. Years earlier, with support from the National Cancer Institute, Giovanella had gathered breast tumors soon after they were removed from patients. He broke them up and implanted them under the skin of "nude mice," hairless laboratory animals with deficient immune systems that do not reject human or other foreign tissue. Giovanella's aim was to induce breast-tumor growth that would continue through successive mouse generations so that he might study the tumors over time. He implanted 227 tumors, of which only 16 took and grew, and each of those 16 came from women whose cancer had been especially aggressive and almost always fatal. Giovanella sent Slamon samples of 11 of the tumors, and Slamon determined that 7 of them overexpressed Her-2/neu. Over the next year, Giovanella and Slamon injected samples of the antibody into mice with tumors that overexpressed the gene, and the tumors shrank. He observed no effect on the mice whose tumors did not overexpress Her-2/neu.

Other labs offered further proof that Her-2/neu could make a normal cell cancerous. Philip Leder at Harvard Medical School bred a strain of mice that overexpressed Her-2/neu from birth and developed breast cancer at an especially high rate. He found that their tumors could be treated successfully with the antibody.

Now Slamon's enthusiasm exploded. These were not cells growing in a dish or even mouse tumors. These were human breast cancers growing in mice, and the antibody stopped the cancerous growth. Slamon remembers phoning Ullrich to share his excitement. "This is as close as we're going to get to testing in humans without actually using humans," Slamon said.

By 1988, it was clear to Slamon and the team at Genentech that they were working with a promising new therapy for the treatment of breast and, as it turned out, ovarian cancers. (Slamon had found Her-2/neu overexpression in about 20 percent of ovarian cancers.) One might assume that an experiment in which four or five scientists were producing results of such enormous potential would have immediately attracted Genentech's attention. But potential alone does not guarantee the corporate green light. The company owned the rights to the antibody, but at that time it had set itself on a strategic course that did not include investing in cancer treatments of any sort. Not that the company didn't see the need and the market for new gene-based cancer treatments. But it had tried and failed and had no wish to pour additional money into a hopeless enterprise. Frustrated by many things, including Genentech's refusal to invest in developing Her-2/neu further, Ullrich quit, started his own company in California, and took a major professorship in Germany.

From the first, Genentech's young managers shared the can-do attitude of its scientists. The company headquarters looks like a huge college campus. Casual dress is de rigueur; ties are nowhere to be seen, and big Friday-afternoon beer bashes were a crucial part of the company's culture. To celebrate its twentieth anniversary, the company displayed a banner modeled on the cover of the Beatles' *Sergeant Pepper* album, with pictures of company bigwigs in band uniforms surrounded by well-known figures ranging from Charles Darwin to Ronald Reagan. "Lean and mean" was the credo. Let the pharmaceutical giants employ huge bureaucracies and execute research and development based on incomprehensible flowcharts. Genentech's decisions would often follow gut instinct and hunches, a management style that a Genentech veteran who now works at another company describes as "often completely and totally screwy." In the words of John Curd, a medical director, who came on board in 1991, "Management would hear four or five presentations and say, 'This sounds great. I like this one.' And we were off."

With its pioneer mentality, Genentech quickly encountered the harsh reality that soon shattered many of the early fantasies of the biotechnology industry. If a high-tech start-up invents a revolutionary new chip, it can almost sell it the next morning. But no matter how promising a drug appears in the laboratory or even in animals, it must undergo years of staggeringly expensive clinical trials before anyone really knows whether it works. So a mistake in judgment about what to test in clinical trials can set a company on the wrong course for years and eat up tens—even hundreds—of millions of dollars.

As Genentech matured from its arrogant youth into the adult real world of drug development, it coped by splitting its corporate personality in half. The science remained excellent. Genentech researchers continued to attend meetings where they talked openly about their work; they continued to publish in the best journals. But no matter what the early dreams, those scientists would never be the people who actually tested, or certainly ever sold, drugs. The managers hired for these tasks faced enormous pressure and at times resorted to disreputable tactics. Allegations emerged about stock payoffs to academic researchers who were supposed to render unbiased judgments in clinical trials. There were hints about highly suspect marketing schemes that included threatening doctors with malpractice suits if they did not prescribe a Genentech product. Genentech gained a dual reputation as a center of great science and sleazy business. As Art Levinson, a veteran Genentech research scientist who became CEO in 1995, put it: "We have always had fun, but we haven't always been proud to work here."

In its early years, Genentech had invested heavily in reputed cancer elixirs called interferons, proteins that regulate the immune system. Genentech tested those drugs not so much because they had reliable leads from good, solid science but because the claim that interferons could cure cancer had captured the public's attention. In the early years of biotechnology the accompanying hype attracted capital. *Time* magazine put interferon on its cover ("The Big If"), and other mainstream news organizations touted its supposed cancer-curing properties. In fact, there are several different interferons, but at the start, it was seen as a singular panacea.

This enthusiasm for interferon was largely due to the efforts of one individual, Mathilda Krim, a Swiss-born biochemist working at Sloan Kettering in New York. Krim was a masterful promoter, unequaled at the art of molding both scientific and public opinion. Years later she made an invaluable contribution to the fight against AIDS by joining forces with Elizabeth Taylor to establish the American Foundation for AIDS Research.

By the mid-1970s, the War on Cancer seemed to be faltering, at least in the eyes of the public and politicians. Krim stepped in to reinvigorate the campaign. "The American Cancer Society and some of the others felt they would really like to have something dramatic happen," she said later. "They wanted something that went 'whammo' against cancer." Without substantial evidence that interferon actually worked, Krim set about convincing the public that it was a cure, mobilizing all her connections and considerable charm. Her husband, Arthur Krim—a former chairman of United Artists, cofounder of Orion Pictures, and a major force in Democratic politics—was instrumental in winning her access to political and media heavyweights. She threw receptions at her posh Manhattan townhouse, mixing scientists working on interferon with a hand-picked group of influential figures ranging from Anwar Sadat to Woody Allen. With surprisingly little hard evidence, the public and even certain scientists began to buy into the hype that interferon was a cure for cancer. Genentech's leaders followed suit.

The impulsiveness had a price. Genentech's clinical trials for alpha interferon revealed that it was not, as hoped, a treatment for a broad range of cancers. It turned out to be effective only with a rare type called hairy-cell leukemia—hardly destined to be a profit center for the company. Genentech subsequently licensed the rights to alpha interferon to Hoffman–La Roche, which eventually found a large market for the drug as a treatment for hepatitis B and Kaposi's sarcoma, the AIDS-related skin cancer. Two other products, gamma interferon and a related chemical called TNF, proved to be even less useful, costing Genentech hundreds of millions of dollars.

Burned by the interferon trials, Genentech disbanded its clinical-trial oncology staff and gave up on cancer. By the time the company brass had to decide whether to take Her-2/neu to the next stage, human trials, there was little enthusiasm. Genentech's profits were coming primarily from Activase, or t-PA, which dissolves blood clots that cause heart attacks, and human growth factor, used to help prevent dwarfism in children. "They were really very allergic to cancer," according to Mike Shepard, who joined Genentech straight out of graduate school, just about the time of the initial public offering in 1980. He took over the Her-2 laboratory program when Ullrich left.

Shepard, who wears pop-bottle-thick glasses and has a tonsure surrounded by blond hair, is an exuberant man who tends to shout rather than talk, speaks in hyperbole, and waves his hands for emphasis. The Her-2/neu program, he says, was a blueprint for the proper biotech method. "First you understand the molecular events that give rise to a dangerous cancer. Then you look at that pathway, and based on technology that you have in your hands right now, you design in your head a treatment." He believed he had a molecule that could treat breast and ovarian cancers. He kept trying to get approval from senior management to move ahead, but never got it.

What Shepard perceived as the continual rejection exacted a huge toll on him and his staff. Despite the freedom to pursue one's own research interest, success in the company still depended on having the research converted to a clinical treatment. "In order to make a product like this successful," he says, "people actually give up their careers. They have nervous breakdowns, and they don't survive in this field. They just can't cope with the company saying no." One man in his group, "a brilliant young scientist," got so fed up that he left the field altogether and went to law school, an act that Shepard equates with creating "human debris."

While Shepard was fighting for the Her-2/neu program from within, Slamon was making a pest of himself from without. His research efforts, effectively his whole life, now focused completely on the effort to make a drug out of the antibody. He did not want to hear that Genentech had no interest in his treatment for breast cancer. He tirelessly phoned company executives and flew up to San Francisco to confront them. Like the most tenacious Washington lobbyist, he worked the Genentech hallways, cajoling the senior management group, which the younger scientists had dubbed the village elders, to give life to Her-2/neu research.

"Long before we got into development, Denny was here. I mean, Denny would go talk to everybody that was in senior management," recalls John Curd, a manager who approaches his work with a keen-eyed skepticism. "He had a way of talking to people and convincing them, charming them, that, yeah, this was an important project." Slamon recalls that his message was always the same: "You've got something real here. If you don't want to make it, license it out. I'll go find somebody that'll produce enough of the protein that we can put it into patients. Someone should at least take a critical look at the data."

No one questioned Slamon's near religious faith in Her-2, but many considered his full-court press on Genentech quixotic. Not only did he not own the rights to the antibody, but also he had no money and almost no professional reputation to bank on. "Here's a guy who was pushing a scientific concept and using a pharmaceutical company to develop a drug because he knew that he couldn't develop the drug himself," says Curd. "I can tell you, his input into Her-2 early and his championship of the product both in his lab and his own personal resources and at Genentech was unrivaled. Nobody gave a shit except him." The Her-2 effort went nowhere for a year and a half and seemed headed for oblivion.

A company's decision to proceed with the clinical development of a drug is always a source of tension, part of what the biotechnology world calls normal pharma business. Scientists invariably believe their idea will pan out while the company officials in clinical affairs, ever aware of the staggering costs and risks of human trials, regard the researchers as starry-eyed idealists whose exuberance must be contained. So it was not uncommon at Genentech, especially with its chaotic management style, for many projects to teeter on the brink of extinction and, consequently, for scientists like Mike Shepard—and Axel Ullrich before him—to feel scorned.

Genentech management had plenty of reason to worry that the treatment would not work. The antibody—then known as 4D5—that Mike Shepard and Dennis Slamon had worked on in their labs was a kind of monoclonal antibody, that is, a pure solution of an antibody that attacks a single target. But all monoclonal antibodies are developed from genes in mice or other laboratory animals. Thus the Her-2/neu antibody that Shepard was cloning was a mouse protein. Ever since scientists started creating monoclonal antibodies in the mid-1970s, they had theorized that these antibodies would constitute the long-sought-after "magic bullets" that would either destroy rogue cells or transport a poison to carry out selective cellular assassination. Scientists and venture capitalists set up biotechnology companies with those very missions. But the monoclonals' mouse origins nearly proved their undoing.

When the human immune system encounters a protein from another species, it responds by producing antibodies to attack the intruder in the same way it demolishes invading bacteria. This immune response gets stronger with every exposure. So a human might tolerate one dose of a mouse antibody, but the second, third, and fourth doses provoke a massive reply from the immune system, obliterating the antibodies long before they reach the cancer they are meant to attack. Occasionally, the response can trigger an allergic reaction severe enough to threaten a patient's life.

Another potential pitfall stood in the way of using antibodies to treat cancer. Antibodies often made their targets on cancer cells disappear—a phenomenon known in molecular biology as "down-regulation." It would quickly render any treatment useless. It is tempting to think of the cell's surface as a fixed landscape, such as the side of mountain. But in reality it is more like the surface of a pot of boiling water, where the molecules, like bubbles, appear, then disappear in an instant. And once antibodies attack a particular cancer, their molecular target on the cell surface often vanishes, and the cancer continues to grow out of control.

The thinking behind some biotech companies was that a single magic-bullet treatment could successfully fight cancer. But all attempts had failed. The biotech companies that were set up to hurl monoclonals at cancer and other diseases either moved on to different treatments or failed outright. Aware of these experiences, many of Genentech's village elders reacted to the proposal to use the Her-2/neu antibody with near derision. Everyone knew monoclonal antibodies would never work against cancer.

In mid-1989, management almost shut down the Her-2 project. Two scientists in lower management came to the rescue. David Botstein, a prominent molecular biologist who had served three years as vice president for research, and Art Levinson, a cancer researcher who had helped Ullrich clone the Her-2/neu gene and was moving up through management ranks, both believed, despite the popular wisdom, that antibodies had a future in medical care. Neither was certain that Her-2 would be the antibody to prove their belief, but they argued their case and won a stay of execution for the laboratory research so that the clinical trial would remain a possibility.

Finally, in late 1989, Her-2 found its champion in top management. Bill Young was a vice president for manufacturing and a village elder, a member of the committee that made key decisions about product development. His interaction with the research scientists was minimal, and like the others in the inner circle he had been leery of getting sucked into another financial black hole to support a cancer therapy. Then his mother developed metastatic breast cancer.

He learned how few effective treatments were available to women suffering from this virulent form of the disease. "I got very interested in what Genentech could be doing," Young recalls. "I was wandering around Research [the company's laboratories] one day and ran into Mike Shepard, who was at that time working on Her-2." The scientists were pushing for development support, but management just hadn't been interested. Now Young was interested, and Shepard asked Slamon to fly up and meet with him. "We started talking about it, and we cooked up the idea that there's a good way of pursuing this," says Young. "This is a potential nontoxic therapy that could really work for women." From then on, when ad hoc management committees met to consider the Her-2 project, Young offered enthusiastic support for proceeding with human tests.

Genentech presented itself to investors as a sophisticated corporation that had outgrown the rashness of an upstart and made rational decisions based on sound business principles. But the truth was that passionate interest in a project, especially from someone with a voice in the financial decisions, was critical to the equation. "Although we do all that we can to be very logical about the projects that we carry forward—we analyze them and have our data in hand and know the markets and probabilities—it still takes someone in the company to be very interested in a project to make it go forward," explains Young. "And it's usually got to be a management person [who] gets interested in what's happening and helps shepherd that project through the early stages, which are usually the most formative and which [are] where things easily get killed."

Bill Young, a man whose mother was dying of breast cancer, persuaded his fellow elders that the antibody, despite all the reasons for doubt, might be a genuine cancer breakthrough, that it was worth the company's investment of resources. Just like that, one man flipped the switch on Her-2.

CHAPTER 4

Courting the Thought Leader

enentech's sudden and unpredicted decision in late 1989 to pursue Her-2/neu changed everything for Mike Shepard and his dejected team. Once marginalized, they found themselves sought after and became vital contributors to decision making as Genentech took the drug into the complex and expensive process of development. Always aware that the village elders could change their minds unexpectedly, Shepard moved as fast as possible.

Genentech, however, had a new card in its deck to try to overcome the antibodies' mouse origins. Along with a few other companies, it had begun testing a promising new technology. It had recently hired Paul Carter, an agonizingly shy twenty-nine-year-old Englishman who had learned how to "humanize" monoclonal antibodies at the Medical Research Council Laboratories in Cambridge, England. The goal was to make the biological equivalent of a wolf in sheep's clothing, that is, a mouse protein that the human body would recognize as a human protein.

Antibodies are large proteins, and like all proteins their attributes are coded by genes, the specific stretches of DNA made up of the bases represented by the letters A, C, T, and G. To perform the biotech wizardry of humanizing the mouse version of an antibody, Carter started with the two genes that carry the code for the mouse monoclonal antibody. He then reached into his library of genes that carry the code for human antibodies and replaced most of the sequence of As, Cs, Ts, and Gs in the mouse genes with sequences from human genes. The newly created genes then produced a new protein, the humanized antibody. The only part of the new protein that remained murine—or mouse—in origin was the tiny but critical section where the antibody binds to its target.

The hope was that the humanized antibody would still attach to the Her-2/neu molecules on the surface of cancer cells without provoking an immune response. Theoretically, the humanization process made sense, but no one knew if it would work. When Carter set out to humanize the Her-2/neu antibody in 1990, only two people in the world had received injections of humanized antibodies. Both were patients with non-Hodgkin's lymphoma. A humanized antibody directed against the cancer caused the tumors of both patients to shrink and elicited no immune response. The experiments were successful, but two cases hardly provide confidence in a new therapy.

For the last two months of 1989, Shepard and his colleagues worked around the clock to clone the antibody genes so that Carter could create the humanized version. It was a painstaking task. "The company had not yet made a full commitment," Shepard says. "But once we had cloned the antibody genes, [it] would hardly be a good time to kill the project. So we pushed ahead." Shepard gave Carter the genes just after the new year.

Soon after that, Genentech lost its innocence. On February 2, 1990, Roche Holding, Ltd., a Swiss company that owns Hoffmann-La Roche, agreed to pay $2.1 billion for 60 percent of Genentech's stock and picked up an option to buy the remainder over several years. Economic necessity had forced the move. Like other biotechnology companies, Genentech was constantly starved for cash. When Roche took over, Genentech had only two drugs on the market: human growth hormone, which was never a big seller, and t-PA, the clot dissolver used to treat heart attacks. Genentech's leaders assumed that t-PA would bring in most of the company's profits. But the company was choking on the financial fallout of studies showing that t-PA, which sold for $2,000 a dose, was no better than a competing drug that sold for one tenth the price.

Some members of Genentech's rabidly aggressive sales force tried to overcome the obstacle by spreading false information about its competitor's product and trying to persuade physicians that the studies were flawed. Genentech even recruited nurses working in cardiology units to act as sales representatives during their shifts to try and convince doctors of t-PA's usefulness. The company ran seminars where lawyers hinted that doctors might face malpractice suits if they failed to prescribe t-PA. Subsequent studies would show t-PA to be slightly better than its lower-priced competitor, but sales fell far below what the company had promised investors. Genentech's leaders faced the prospect of a hostile takeover in which they would lose control if they did not negotiate a friendly acquisition that left the power in their hands.

Robert Swanson, Genentech's CEO, negotiated the buyout, working with Kirk Raab, who became Genentech's president in 1985. Age forty-nine at the time of the deal, Raab had worked his way up the sales divisions of several pharmaceutical companies and was president of Abbott Laboratories before joining Genentech. Many stock analysts warmly greeted Genentech's decision to hire Raab as a sign that the brash young company was finally reaching out for expertise from the pharmaceutical industry. But Raab soon took over completely. When the Roche deal was completed, Swanson left Genentech to return to the venture-capital firm where he had worked when he created Genentech. Swanson said his departure was voluntary. But many news accounts made it clear that Raab had won a power struggle.

Swanson, the venture capitalist and visionary who had cofounded Genentech when he was just twenty-seven, had been the soul of Genentech, nurturing the freedom for its scientists along with the gung-ho company culture. Raab, who also took over as CEO when Swanson left, was a smooth corporate type, more interested in sales than in science. Even in the face of financial reality, Genentech's employees were resentful. Their leaders had sold out to one of the hated behemoths. Swanson had always told anyone who would listen that Genentech would never be sold, that it would mature into an integrated pharmaceutical company. Years after the deal, scientists at Genentech could still be seen wearing T-shirts bearing the fictional *San Francisco Chronicle* headline GENENTECH BUYS ROCHE. It was the kind of takeover they had dreamed of.

Shortly after the buyout, Jürgen Drews, Roche's president of international research and development and a new member of Genentech's board of directors, arrived in South San Francisco to meet with Genentech's senior scientists. "He didn't like antibodies," Shepard remembers. "So he wasn't very excited about Her-2/neu." When Roche cut Shepard's lab budget, the end seemed to be at hand yet again. But Genentech's senior management continued its support, perhaps to test Roche's promises of independence. Bill Young continued to be a booster, as was Art Levinson, who was by then a senior vice president. But years of competition for steps up the corporate ladder had left their mark. Others in the company say Levinson, from research division, and Young, from manufacturing, don't get along. For the record both deny any rift. But others say that Her-2's two biggest boosters in senior management never spoke to each other unless it was absolutely necessary.

Despite the budget cuts, Shepard, with eager backing from Bill Young, managed to persuade Genentech management to spend $3 million for Dennis Slamon to test the mouse antibody in human volunteers while everyone waited for the humanized version from

Paul Carter. The experiment was certainly questionable. The mouse antibody itself would never become a drug and could provoke a dangerous immune response—so dangerous that neither Slamon nor Genentech would risk giving any patient more than one dose. But the experiment might determine whether the whole idea of using Her-2/neu was simply wrong. Although Her-2/neu is overexpressed only on cancer cells, the gene itself resides in many different cells in the human body. Using the mouse antibody, Slamon might establish that the treatment would not cause the body some terrible harm by attacking noncancerous cells. Slamon and Shepard also attached radioactive atoms to the antibody so that they could track its progress and see if it actually found its way to the cancer it was supposed to attack.

Before beginning the human testing, Genentech paid for an outside lab to inject the mouse antibody in dogs, rats, and monkeys (small companies typically contract out such routine testing). When those tests revealed no evidence of toxicity, the next step was to prove that the concept of antibody treatment was sound. Genentech produced enough mouse antibody for Slamon to inject twenty women with highly advanced cancers, half breast cancers, half ovarian. In every case, the cancerous cells overexpressed Her-2/neu. After years of rejection, Shepard's Her-2/neu team was finally going to test the mouse version of the drug in human patients.

In the spring of 1990, Diane Hinton, a thirty-one-year-old mother of three boys then aged thirteen, eleven, and ten, was in the midst of a losing battle with ovarian cancer. One day, her mother came across a tiny item in the business section of *The Sacramento Bee* reporting that Genentech was moving a promising breast- and ovarian-cancer treatment into advanced development. It took her two days to reach Slamon by telephone, and he referred her daughter to an oncologist at UCLA who was screening volunteers. Diane

Hinton, barely five feet tall and weighing eighty-five pounds, was invited to join the trial. She and her husband, Scott, left their house in Hanford, near Fresno, to drive to Los Angeles.

Of course, there was never the slightest chance that the mouse antibody would help Diane Hinton or the other volunteers. But like most patients in early-phase cancer-drug trials, she ignored the warnings on the consent form and signed it. She had volunteered for Slamon's experiment hoping for some magic that would save her life. A *Los Angeles Times Magazine* article in October 1991 described how Hinton and the nineteen other women spent four days being poked and prodded and photographed for the benefit of science.

After taking half an hour to explain the experiment to Diane and her adoring husband, Slamon sat back, crossed his arms against his chest, and studied the couple. "You know," he said finally, shaking his head, "I really don't understand why people would voluntarily take a drug that might kill them. You two have some quality time left. Yet you're giving us a week of that time. As far as I'm concerned, you're the real heroes here." Said Diane, "We feel this is my last chance." "We don't feel like heroes," added Scott.

In the face of impossible odds, Hinton never lost her sense of humor. At one point during the trial, she conspired with the nurses to deliver a message to Slamon saying that she had suffered a reaction to the antibody. When he burst into her room, he found his patient lying in bed wearing a mouse mask.

In fact, the tests showed that the mouse antibody produced no toxic reaction. Later on, Genentech management would argue that the trial could have proved little else because there was no chance that Slamon could give any of the patients more than one dose. Despite the overwhelming odds, Slamon does not rule out the possibility that the mouse antibody may actually have helped Diane Hinton: "I can tell you that she was supposed to be dead by Christmas of that year, and she lived for another three years." She died in 1993.

Paul Carter's efforts to humanize the antibody succeeded brilliantly. He accomplished the feat in ten months. "I think what really amazed everybody at Genentech was the speed with which he did it," says Hank Fuchs, a researcher who would later play a big role in the program. "The speed and precision—it was a sensational piece of work." In fact, laboratory experiments revealed that one of the new antibodies Carter created bound more tightly to its target than the original mouse antibody had. Another set of animal tests showed the humanized version to be nontoxic.

Despite the encouraging news, not everyone at Genentech was enthusiastic. John Curd, who joined Genentech in 1991, does not hide his disdain for the way Genentech pursued Her-2/neu and other treatments. "There was unbridled enthusiasm that some of these scientific ideas or biologic ideas would work," he says.

Curd, a native of Gunnison, Colorado, attended Princeton and Harvard Medical School. He spent most of his career in the academic atmosphere of the Scripps Clinic and Research Foundation in La Jolla before moving to Genentech as a medical director at age forty-six. Surgery for a benign brain tumor in 1996 slightly hampered Curd's speech. But neither the operation nor the corporate culture in which he found himself restrained Curd from speaking his mind—a trait that often evoked the wrath of his bosses.

"Genentech's changed a lot, and I would tell you that in ninety-one, people's concept of drug development was much less developed than it is today," Curd says. Based on simple business principles, he believed that Her-2/neu's potential would never justify the crushing cost—ultimately more than $150 million—of getting the drug to market. Because a minority of breast-cancer patients—25 to 30 percent—suffer from the type of disease positively affected by the treatment, "today if Her-2 came forward, you couldn't get it into development," he says. If the decision had been his, Genentech would never have taken Her-2/neu to advanced development. But when he arrived, the company was already committed to developing Her-2/neu.

Curd had little choice but to assist the company's efforts to win FDA approval of the drug. He decided that the treatment should be tested only against breast cancer because the tumors associated with it are easier to measure than those of other cancers, a critical requirement because measurable tumor growth or shrinkage is a reliable index of a disease's response to treatment. He eliminated ovarian cancer from the trials because in its advanced stages the disease generally appears as a diffuse mass throughout the abdomen. When the drug won approval for breast cancer, he reasoned, testing for ovarian cancer would quickly follow.

For Curd, the next crucial decision was where to carry out the human tests. Drug trials consist of three parts: phase I monitors the treatment for side effects and establishes the correct dosages; phase II makes the first foray into understanding the treatment's possible effectiveness. If phase I reveals no unexpected problem, the testing usually flows without problem into phase II. The first two phases typically enroll a few dozen patients. Phase III is a wholly different process. It is a test with hundreds, even thousands of patients to establish whether the drug works well enough to support an application to the FDA to bring it to market.

All three phases are carried out under the eye of the FDA, which is empowered to grant final approval. Only a few academic medical centers have the capability to carry out phase I and II trials for possible cancer drugs. They must have experienced staffs and extensive facilities to monitor volunteers—usually patients with advanced disease and no other options left—for a broad range of side effects. They must also keep detailed records for the FDA. Doctors who are faculty members in teaching hospitals actively seek phase I and II studies to further their careers and to promote their institutions. To potential patients, a medical center carrying

out the early studies offers the latest and most experimental therapies—a strong selling point for many desperate cancer patients.
For doctors, early-phase trials give access to the latest treatments
and afford opportunities to publish and to build their reputa-
tions—critical steps to advancing their academic careers.

Curd wanted to conduct the Her-2/neu phase I trials at two or
three institutions in order to foster competition in enrolling volunteers. In trials, the rule is that the doctor whose institution enrolls
the most volunteers wins the right to be senior author of the published paper explaining the results. Dennis Slamon had already set
up a network of oncologists throughout southern California who
would refer patients to him. He believed he could attract enough
patients to carry out most, if not all, of the phase I and II trials.

Curd did everything in his power to keep Slamon from running
the show, despite his role in the early development. "I admire
Dennis Slamon for manipulating Genentech into developing
Her-2/neu," Curd says. "The drug became his scientific raison
d'être. Now once it becomes clear that the drug has activity and
value, other people get involved with different expertise. I don't
think Denny Slamon's knowledge of breast cancer is probably the
best in the country."

Curd's strategy was to win the cooperation of a doctor who was
universally regarded as a leader in the field of breast-cancer treatment: Larry Norton, head of the breast-cancer service at Sloan
Kettering. Curd considers Norton "a thought leader," a physician
whose ideas, attitudes, and prescribing habits influence hundreds
of others in the field. Without Norton's participation, Curd believed a new breast-cancer treatment held little chance of success
or acceptance.

But he recalls the challenge of trying to win Norton over in
1992: "When you went out to talk to people like Larry Norton
about Her-2, they didn't have time to talk to you. I mean they were

kind of interested. But their concept is 'Nontoxic biologics don't work. Antibodies don't work. Next case.' " At the time, Norton believed passionately in the power of chemotherapy.

Norton grew up in Brooklyn and Long Island. His father, Morley, writing under the name Morley Post, wrote the travel column for the *New York Post*. Norton trained with a giant in chemotherapy, Emil "Tom" Frei III, a disciple of Sidney Farber's. While working as a researcher for the National Cancer Institute in 1977, Norton helped develop a mathematical model that he says still forms the basis of his approach to cancer treatment. He explains it using the metaphor of crabgrass in a garden: "When the whole garden's filled with crabgrass, almost anything you do in terms of killing [it] is going to have a dramatic impact. And you're going to say, 'My God, I'm accomplishing something.' But getting rid of the last few plants is very difficult, as every gardener knows." Fighting cancer is comparable: only a very heavy dose of chemotherapy will rid the body of the last cancer cells. Norton firmly believes in the highest possible doses—if bone-marrow transplants or pain and suffering are involved, so be it. The goal, he reasons, is to save lives.

Among patients, especially the wealthy and well connected in New York, Norton enjoys a reputation as the dispenser of the best, most advanced care available for breast cancer. The significance of winning an appointment to see him is perhaps best described by Joyce Wadler in her book *My Breast*. "I have the feeling from what other doctors have told me, that in Breast Cancerland, this is akin to being invited to God's for drinks," she writes.

When Norton sweeps into the examining room, usually late and trailed by an entourage, patients meet a short, thin, bespectacled, bald, middle-aged man with a fringe of gray hair. Supremely self-assured, he scans the room for the expected approval whenever he opens his mouth to dispense his rapid-fire wisdom. Highly articulate and exuding a laser-beam intensity, he is a man who clearly commands, expects, and receives respect. Like Zeus ruling from

Mount Olympus, he is accustomed to deferential treatment. When he's beyond earshot, his staff slyly refers to him as "El Nortino."

Norton also believes that his patients' willingness to accept his aggressive treatment plays a big role in their outcomes. "I can tell right away, almost before we talk, whether the patient is classifiable into [one of] two types," he says. "One of them comes in and says by the way [she] talk[s] and by the way [she] act[s], 'Doctor, whatever you do, don't hurt me. Don't give me bad news. Don't tell me anything that's gonna disturb me. And don't give me any medications or do anything to me that's gonna make me ill.' The other says, 'Doctor, whatever you do, cure me. I'm here to get better. I'm here to win. Tell me what I need to win.' There's no question the patient that comes in and says, 'I'm here to get better'—she's going to do better."

Norton's appeal to patients can be traced in part to his boundless optimism. He is undeterred by statistics showing how little the breast-cancer death rate has improved in the last fifty years. "We can change the natural history of the disease in terms of recurrence-free overall survival. It's extremely exciting, and I really think it ought to be emphasized because" at meetings of scientists "there is a lot of talk about the complexity of the problem of cancer. All right, there's sort of implied pessimism there. And I always like to stand up and say, 'Wait a minute; you've got to understand that you're seeing it from this particular vantage point. I can cure breast cancer right now. I can cure it by surgical intervention. I can cure it with radiation therapy in early-stage cases. I can affect the natural history and cure some people of the disease by giving drugs in the adjuvant setting, and I can dramatically affect the natural history of the disease in the advanced-stage setting as well. Interventions work. What we have to do is make those interventions work better.' "

Norton treated Linda McCartney, wife of ex-Beatle Paul McCartney. She survived less than three years after her diagnosis. In an interview two days after her death in April 1998, Norton maintained his characteristically rosy outlook about breast cancer treatment in general. "We are not curing everybody and for this reason we have to work harder," he said, "but I think the prospects for the future are very promising."

To try to win Norton's support for the Her-2/neu trial, Curd approached Norton's boss, John Mendelsohn, chief of medicine at Sloan Kettering. Mendelsohn was not a breast-cancer specialist, but he lobbied Norton to listen to Curd. Mendelsohn and Curd had been colleagues at the Scripps Clinic where Mendelsohn's research focused on the EGF (epidermal growth factor) receptor, the same molecule that attached to the receptor Axel Ullrich cloned before Her-2/neu. Just as certain breast- and ovarian-cancer cells overexpress Her-2/neu, cells in several types of cancer overexpress the EGF receptor; Mendelsohn was trying to find an antibody to treat those cancers. He was one of the few research physicians who really thought antibodies would ever play a role in fighting cancer. Norton, on the other hand, was extremely skeptical of antibodies, but he agreed to give them a try because of Mendelsohn.

Curd also won the cooperation of Craig Henderson, the head of oncology at the University of California, San Francisco, who had extensive experience with clinical trials. As the field's most vocal opponent of high-dose chemotherapy with bone-marrow transplant, he was seeking alternatives to chemotherapy. He, too, was skeptical of antibodies, but they intrigued him all the same.

Henderson passed the bulk of the day-to-day work to Debu Tripathey, a young medical scientist who had studied Her-2/neu at MIT. At Sloan Kettering, Norton similarly deputized José Baselga, a research fellow from Barcelona.

At UCLA, Curd allowed Slamon to conduct just part of the phase I trials, and as they progressed, he would further diminish Slamon's role. By wooing oncologists like Norton, whose treatment philosophy differed radically from Slamon's, he set up a rivalry that colored the entire course of the clinical trials. Slamon deeply resented Norton's involvement and can barely hide his contempt for hosannas tossed in the doctor's direction. Slamon believed Norton's enthusiasm for chemotherapy was misplaced. He saw the treatment's results day in and day out, and he called it the hand-grenade approach—throwing in poisons and hoping "you kill more bad cells than good cells."

In reality, Norton embraced whatever treatment appeared most promising at any particular moment. A large part of his success stemmed from his ability not just to move with the tide of medical opinion but to remain slightly ahead of it. Norton is a "thought leader" precisely because he manages to remain both authoritative and open to new ideas, giving him the power to shift conventional wisdom.

Slamon, of course, used the best treatments for his patients, but his overriding goal was to pluck out the one big nugget—the treatment he developed. As Slamon put it, "When you go up to the window and place a bet you can't ask for a ticket on the horse that is going to win. You have to pick one."

A Fabulous Endowment

ven as Genentech was trying to minimize his role in the trials, Slamon's stature outside the company was growing. Because of one particular patient, money was no longer a problem for him. In 1982, as he was finishing up his clinical training at UCLA, he had gotten a call from a medical-school friend asking him to take on a new patient, Brandon Tartikoff. Tartikoff was desperately ill four years after undergoing treatment for Hodgkin's disease. As with most other cancers, a recurrence of Hodgkin's disease poses a greater threat than the initial appearance.

Tartikoff had changed the face of American television. Touted as NBC's boy genius of programming, he would soon catapult the network from its seemingly perpetual number-three ranking to the top of the ratings with hits like *Cheers* and *The Cosby Show*. Only thirty years old, he was beginning his third year as head of entertainment at NBC, the youngest person ever to hold that powerful position. When the most recent symptoms appeared, his internist diagnosed him with a recurrence of Hodgkin's. Slamon had been reluctant to see Tartikoff. "You know, I'm seeing general oncology patients. I'm just finishing up my fellowship, so I'm not the most senior person," he remembers telling his friend. But he felt confident that he could handle a simple case of Hodgkin's disease.

Slamon found his new patient formidable yet very likable. "I'm just starting as a junior attending. And I know a little about this guy, in the sense that NBC is in the cellar but is starting to make its move with some new programming, and he's in the paper all the time," he says. "He's got a great sense of humor, and he had a great sense of humor even about this." Slamon prescribed an experimental and aggressive course of chemotherapy.

Enter Lilly Tartikoff, described by more than one acquaintance as "a force of nature." Tall in stature and with prominent cheekbones, a finely pointed chin and nose, and a lithe body—a testament to her days as a ballet dancer—she was on her way to becoming one of the few Hollywood wives to carve out a presence of her own. She had grown up in Los Angeles and had won a scholarship to the Juilliard School in New York. From there, she made it into the illustrious corps de ballets of George Balanchine's New York City Ballet, and while dancing, she met Brandon. Eventually, injuries stalled her career, and in 1980, at age twenty-six, she moved back to the West Coast to work in her father's accessories business. She married Brandon two years later.

One day soon after Slamon had discussed the combination chemotherapy with Brandon, she called him demanding to know what was happening with her husband. Lilly was not about to put blind faith even in a doctor who, like Slamon, had come highly recommended. "I told him that he was going to have to deal with me, because I was the one who was going to be the caretaker," she says. Slamon asked her if she had talked to her husband, and he explained that as his doctor he was not at liberty to disclose confidential information.

The next day, Lilly showed up at Slamon's office without an appointment. It was quite a scene. "How dare you not tell me what's going on with my husband?" she demanded. Slamon was taken aback and suggested that the three of them meet. When they were all sitting in the same room, Slamon explained that he wanted Brandon to try a particularly powerful course of combination therapy. Lilly asked a lot of questions, and Slamon answered all of them. She remembers how reassuring Slamon was. "It was better than meeting Marcus Welby, MD," she says. Brandon heard him out, then said simply, "I have faith in you. Go ahead and let's try it." As Slamon had warned, Brandon lost his hair and felt nauseated and physically and emotionally depleted. "It was much harder than anybody expected," Lilly admits. "The drugs got Brandon down. They played with his emotional system." For someone like Brandon Tartikoff, who was so determinedly upbeat, the depression was particularly hard to take. Still, he never stopped working.

"It was a wild ride," she continues. "NBC was doing very badly. Every week, we read in the newspapers that they were going to fire him." With Brandon's career at such a seemingly precarious point, the couple decided to keep his fragile condition a secret. "Anyone who heard he had cancer assumed he was going to die because that's how most people react." If word had gotten out, it would have damaged what stability he had achieved for himself and the network. "So I told him, . . . 'I [will] take care of you. I will take care of everything that has to do with the cancer stuff. You go to work. You run the network.' "

And so they proceeded through nine cycles of chemotherapy, which lasted almost a year. Brandon was able to continue working through most of it, but there were times when the side effects left him devastated. It was during this period that their daughter was conceived. Calla was born two weeks early, at a time when the chemotherapy had so eroded Brandon's resistance that a trip to the hospital to see his wife and newborn baby was out of the question; doing so would have left him dangerously exposed to disease.

Brandon's work paid off, and he managed to lead the network to ratings triumph. And despite some difficult moments with chemotherapy, when his blood-cell counts dropped so low that he landed in the hospital delirious with fever, he responded to treatment and went back into remission. He remained healthy for a decade and a half.*

In 1986, two years after he had completed chemotherapy, Brandon returned to see Slamon for a routine checkup. Tests showed that he was still in complete remission. That's when Lilly decided she wanted to give something back to Slamon. As the daughter of a Holocaust survivor, she has a deep belief that one always rewards a good deed. "This was a payback," says Lilly. "I don't like to owe anybody anything. He saved Brandon's life, and this was a payback." At first, she framed the idea in a way that she hoped would spare a shy man like Slamon some embarrassment: she said she wanted to help UCLA. Slamon completely missed the tacit message that she wanted to launch his career into orbit. But Lilly was not about to let Slamon's momentary obtuseness discourage her. She started asking him about his research. He explained that his work had nothing to do with Hodgkin's disease; it was in the area of breast cancer. By then, he had discovered the Her-2/neu oncogene. As Slamon remembers it, Lilly said, "I don't care what it's in. If it's new research that's likely to change people's lives, like some research did for Brandon, I want to get behind that."

It is not unheard of for physicians, especially senior academics, to accept donations from wealthy patients for their hospital or research program. The practice is especially common in cancer treatment, where grateful survivors often feel they owe their lives

---

* In 1991, Brandon Tartikoff resigned from NBC to become head of Paramount Pictures. The same year, an automobile accident left the Tartikoffs' daughter permanently disabled. Brandon quit the studio and tried running his own book-publishing and entertainment-production companies. Finally, Hodgkin's disease claimed his life in 1997.

to their oncologist. But Slamon was not a senior faculty member. Furthermore, he now counted the Tartikoffs as his friends. "In the process of treating him and meeting her, you don't have the option of keeping your distance," he says. "They just engage you. They draw you in." The Slamons' daughter, Joey Lyn, is the same age as Calla Tartikoff, and the two girls often played together. Despite Lilly's persistence, he did not want to take advantage of the Tartikoffs' generosity and continued to put off her offers of financial aid. "You don't want to play off that friendship in the setting of having somebody do fund-raising for you," he says. "I always told Lilly, 'No. Your only obligation here is to pay [your] bills.' "

After several years of Slamon's demurrals, Tartikoff tried a new gambit. She called him up in 1989 and said, "I'm sick of this no, no, no. I'm going to do something in cancer. I'm not just doing it for you; I'm doing it because I believe in this research thing, and here's something that's going to convince you." She then issued an ultimatum: if Slamon said no once more, she'd do her fund-raising for Armand Hammer. Hammer, then ninety-one years old and chairman of Occidental Petroleum Corporation, was a controversial figure in business (he had questionable dealings in the Soviet Union, Libya, and other countries hostile to American interests) and medicine. Desperate to cure his own recurrent cancer, he had donated millions of dollars to the Republican Party during the Reagan era to win the chairmanship of the National Cancer Advisory Board, the citizens group that advises the government on cancer-research spending. Flying around the world in his commercial-size private jet, he sought out new and often controversial cancer treatments. One of his pet projects was the highly experimental work of Dr. Steven Rosenberg, chief of surgery at the National Cancer Institute, in immune-based therapies. Cancer researchers held a mixed view of Rosenberg's work, but there was no question that Hammer's attention brought him plenty of publicity and funding. Slamon didn't believe Rosenberg's research needed any more money, so he finally decided to accept Tartikoff's offer. "If you're going to work for cancer anyway," he told her, "then it's a sale."

By this time, Tartikoff's philanthropic contacts included business leaders with financial clout and star power to rival that of Armand Hammer. Earlier in 1989, she was invited to join an advisory board at Max Factor, the cosmetics company now owned by billionaire Ronald Perelman, who also owns Revlon. The board was composed mostly of Hollywood wives who gave the company advice on makeup colors and products. "In the ballet, I wore Max Factor pancake, and I thought, 'OK, that's like a tie-in to my old life,'" says Tartikoff. One day, she was looking at some magazine advertisements for Max Factor products and noticed that the models in the ads were several years older than the teenagers whose interest they were supposed to attract. She wrote a letter to Perelman, whom she'd never met, saying, in effect, "If you want to sell to teenagers, then use models their age."

Perelman, known as one of the shrewdest businessmen in America, knew a smart idea when it landed on his desk. He looked at the Max Factor ads and realized that Tartikoff was absolutely right. He immediately phoned her and offered her a job. She declined. "I have this big life," she said, "and I can't take a full-time job." The following week, she was having lunch at Spago, the popular West Hollywood restaurant, and there was Ronald Perelman eating with a mutual friend. They agreed to get together the next time he was in town. Having at last persuaded Slamon to allow her to raise money for his research, Tartikoff lost no time enlisting Perelman's help. "You're making all this money from women," she lectured him when they got together, "and you should give something back."

Perelman wasn't an easy sell. In the late 1980s, breast cancer still bore something of a social stigma, and the first step was to convince him that it was a better investment of his philanthropic dollars than, say, women in politics, another option then under consideration. It took several meetings in Los Angeles and New York, but Tartikoff brought Perelman around by arguing that a significant contribution to fighting breast cancer would buy him immeasurable goodwill among the people who buy his companies' products. Referring to a dermatology clinic Perelman had financed, Tartikoff told him, "You give millions for zits but nothing for breast cancer." Then she directed his attention to Slamon's work.

She made sure she knew her stuff. Slamon and another oncologist from UCLA, John Glaspy, had spent two afternoons walking her through their research and giving her the essence of her pitch to Perelman. Slamon had had to explain his independent research on Her-2/neu a thousand times and had boiled it down to a simple, effective message: "It's a growth-factor receptor. The more of it you have, the more growth you get. And you can inhibit it with an antibody." Thus armed, Tartikoff met with Perelman and the Revlon board.

In the summer of 1989, Perelman sent Jim Conroy, who oversees the philanthropic activities of Perelman's holding company, MacAndrews and Forbes, out to Los Angeles, as Slamon describes it, "to advise Ronald on whether or not this is something he wants to associate himself with." Conroy, a bearded lawyer with a sharp, streetwise wit, was a bit skeptical but met with Slamon and Glaspy to discuss the research and their needs.

"We get lots and lots of requests," Conroy says. "But I will say that the presentation that this team of doctors made that day really struck me as no other presentation I had heard before or since—both in terms of the kind of radical clarity with which Dennis and his people conceived their research task and the way they formed the questions that they had to answer—and also the sense of urgency that they brought to it—not in a histrionic way, but with a kind of quiet determination about the stakes at play here."

Glaspy's pitch in particular really hit home. The process of receiving money from the National Cancer Institute was so cumbersome that even assuming everything went right, two full years could pass before they got the funding necessary to advance the research. Conroy remembers Glaspy arguing that "in those two years, you've got a Rose Bowl full of women dead from breast cancer. If we had the money to move our research forward and we're right about our hypothesis, we could conceivably save those lives." Conroy asked Slamon, "If we invested in this, how quickly could we move up the time line" for bringing the treatment to patients? Slamon estimated that Revlon's help could speed up the process by three to five years.

That's all Conroy needed to hear. He had been frustrated that Perelman's huge contributions to medicine had not seemed to make a significant impact. "If we're going to put our money someplace, we want to put it where it's likely at least to have a chance of making a move quickly, taking something out of the lab and to the bedside that otherwise wouldn't move that quickly." Here he had finally found a good bet. "[When] something like Her-2/neu has been developed to the point where the infusion of money really makes the difference in terms of advancing the change, that's the dream situation that any foundation likes to come across."

The deal that Lilly Tartikoff and Ronald Perelman made involved a quid pro quo. He would support Slamon's team to the tune of $2.5 million, which immediately made Slamon the best-funded researcher on the UCLA faculty, if she would organize a glittering fund-raiser. The Fire and Ice Ball—an echo of the classic 1952 Revlon advertising campaign for Fire and Ice lipstick—was Perelman's idea. "We had the sense that it would be helpful to have the Los Angeles community in some way put its imprint, its stamp of approval, on our involvement at UCLA," says Conroy. "We're a New York company. And we don't employ a lot of people in Los Angeles. We had no particular relationship to Los Angeles. We wanted to make sure that we were, in fact, endorsed and we were coming in with the approval of the Los Angeles community and would have the community involved in this program, supporting it along with us. We would lead the way, but we wanted to cross the street with everybody."

Tartikoff went at her task with plenty of enthusiasm but little practical knowledge. "I had not raised any money before. I had no experience. I got some bad advice." She saw quickly that in a town like Los Angeles even philanthropic competition is cutthroat. "People are very threatened. It's very political. I said I'm not dealing with any of that. I just made a decision that I was going to raise money and nobody was going to stop me because we were dealing with some vitally important science that was about to break." She brought her undeniable brashness to the enterprise. "I had Brandon's Rolodex," she says. "That meant that I had a history with every one of those people in the Rolodex. Now Brandon had no idea what I was doing. I mean, what I was doing was at times inappropriate and out of line. I was obsessed." She called countless ` people and, in Slamon's words, "harangued" and "harassed" them. When people demurred and pleaded that they had already been generous to other good causes, Tartikoff would ask, "Do you have a wife? Do you have a daughter? Do they have breasts?" Slamon tried to get her to tone down her approach: "I said, 'Lilly, you can't say stuff like this to people.' "

Tartikoff saw herself as Robin Hood. She was aghast at Slamon and Glaspy's working conditions. "They had no money. Dennis had a part-time secretary. I kept saying, 'How can you cure cancer? No one's answering your phones. You're missing phone calls. Your desk is a mess. You're writing grants'—and then there were these huge amounts of money being spent in Hollywood. They'd spend like fifty million dollars on a movie, and when it'd flop, they'd say, 'Oops!' I was guilty of living that life. One of Dennis's graduate students used to ride his bike to work. He was brilliant, but he couldn't afford a car. I kept saying, 'What do you do when it rains?' He'd say, 'I just get wet.' " She was doing what she could to redress this absurd inequity.

Her strong-arm tactics paid off. The first Fire and Ice Ball, a five-hundred-dollar-a-ticket black-tie gala held in March 1990, drew an impressive one thousand guests. If Ronald Perelman had hoped it would establish his presence in Hollywood, it had to have been the night of his dreams. The ballroom at the Beverly Hilton was packed with Hollywood's A list. Among the attendees were the executives Barry Diller and Aaron Spelling, Peter Guber and Michael Eisner. The star power included the likes of Arnold Schwarzenegger, Bob Hope, and Carol Burnett. Naturally, NBC was well represented. The entertainment included the comedian Jay Leno (not yet the host of *The Tonight Show*) and the singers Harry Connick Jr. and Michael Bolton. Addressing the gathering, Lilly Tartikoff promised Slamon, "Now you'll have the backing you deserve." She remembered the actress-comedian Gilda Radner, who had died a year earlier of ovarian cancer. And she thanked her husband, "who taught me there are no limitations." Then she added, "If I've been accused of terrorizing this town, it's his fault." Her fund-raiser grossed $400,000, in addition to the nearly $2.5 million that Revlon had earmarked for Slamon's work.

In the years since 1990, Lilly Tartikoff and Revlon have made the Fire and Ice Ball Los Angeles's premier philanthropic gala. Mel Gibson has emceed, the writer Maya Angelou has offered remarks, and Hillary Rodham Clinton has sent videotaped messages. Barbra Streisand attends regularly. Even in 1997, the year that Brandon Tartikoff lost his battle with Hodgkin's disease, Lilly insisted that the ball go on.

Between 1989 and the end of 1997, Revlon committed more than $13 million to UCLA's work in women's cancers. The Revlon/ UCLA Women's Cancer Research Program, under Slamon's leadership, focused on research, treatment, and educational outreach. As Slamon was bringing in more money than any other UCLA faculty member, the administration decided to make him division chief of oncology and hematology. The administrative duties consumed more and more time. But Slamon, true to the promise, spent most of his time and much of the Revlon money on studies of Her-2/neu. And even though Lilly Tartikoff and Ronald Perleman had no connection to Genentech, both proved to be indispensable allies in the company's efforts to develop and test its drug. Later, Genentech would try to diminish their role, but Hank Fuchs, a key member of Genentech's Her-2 team, said, "Without Denny Slamon and his Revlon money, there would have been no Herceptin."

CHAPTER 6

The First Life Saved

The Revlon money helped Slamon test the mouse antibody on Diane Hinton and the nineteen other volunteers. It also helped him pursue a concept that had struck him just before Genentech decided to forge ahead with the Her-2/neu trials. He wanted to try the antibody in combination with cisplatin, a chemotherapy agent commonly used to treat ovarian and several other cancers. Several studies had shown it to be useless in treating breast cancer, but Slamon had come across other studies on the EGF-receptor antibody that suggested that cisplatin could greatly enhance that antibody's effectiveness. Supported by the Revlon endowment, he confirmed quickly that in the test tube, cisplatin has an enhancing effect on the Her-2/neu antibody as well. With those results in hand, he proposed trying a combination of cisplatin and the Her-2/neu antibody as the best way to treat breast cancer.

Genentech's Her-2/neu team, under Mike Shepard, generated lab results that corroborated Slamon's theory about the cisplatin combination and recommended it to the Genentech management. Genentech embraced the idea wholeheartedly for its first crucial human tests. The company set up phase I and phase II trials at

Sloan Kettering, UCSF, and UCLA to test the antibody alone in women with advanced breast cancer and at UCLA, under Slamon, to test it in combination with cisplatin.

In those tests, the first life was saved by Her-2/neu. Barbara Bradfield, a forty-eight-year-old with a recurrence of breast cancer in her lungs, was on her way to a wellness clinic in Mexico when she got a call from Dennis Slamon. In 1990, when she and her husband, Dean, were on vacation in Big Sur, she had discovered a lump under her arm. Just two months earlier, she had had a clean mammogram, but she knew that a lump under her arm was a bad sign. As soon as she and her husband got back home, she called her doctor. "I had to fight like crazy to get an appointment without waiting for a month," she says. Bradfield, a matronly former schoolteacher whose mild demeanor suggests she would never confront the establishment, was furious. "Finally, when I got really nasty, they worked me in the next day."

In addition to the lump, the doctor found a large mass in her breast. How it had escaped mammography is still a question that nags at her. "Either they missed it in diagnosis, or it grew that fast," she says. "I'm not sure what to think."

Bradfield, a devout Jehovah's Witness, lives in the upscale suburb of La Cañada near Pasadena. Throughout her whole life she never thought about cancer. "There was no breast cancer in my family," she reports. "I spent my life thinking I was somehow some blessed person. Nothing ever went wrong in my life, ever. Just everything I wanted, I got. I mean, that sounds ridiculous, but it's true. I can remember, you know, wanting so badly to be in the Pom-Pom girls in high school, the cheer squad. And when I got that, I thought that was everything, you know, that was so wonderful. And when I went to college and pledged a sorority, I got the sorority I wanted. I mean, it just was everything kind of went my way."

As doctors would later learn, many Her-2/neu-positive breast cancers explode out of nowhere into raging malignancies. Bradfield's friends urged her to pursue a malpractice suit, but she simply didn't have the energy. "You're too absorbed with the other fight," she explains. Doctors judged her cancer to be at stage 3 out of a possible 4, making it a highly life-threatening case, and told her that she had inflammatory breast cancer, which spreads with a terrible virulence. With her daughter Jennifer's help, she started reading up on cancer treatments. In one book, Jennifer found a description of inflammatory breast cancer. "She just got really, really upset because it sounded like there was just no hope," says Bradfield.

Her surgeon sent her to an oncologist in Pasadena. He prescribed a few tests, including one to determine whether the cancer had spread into her bone marrow. Bradfield had heard about the procedure, in which the marrow is extracted from the hip bone with a foot-long needle. "I was scared to death. They put me up on this table and never talked to me." The technician missed the first time he stuck the needle into her leg. When he finally got what he needed, he simply told Bradfield he was finished and instructed her to get dressed. "I got up off the table, and the nerves in my leg were still numb from the test, so I fell," she remembers. "At that moment, I knew what I was dealing with. It was like that experience made the whole thing sink in."

Indeed, Bradfield was terrified, but she was also furious. "I hated the man," she says with a vehemence that for her is not usual. "I mean, I cried all the way through. It's a good thing my husband was with me because he could sit and listen to what the guy was telling me in the room. I didn't hear a thing from that moment on. But then I started searching 'cause I knew I couldn't work with that person.

"I knew I had cancer, and I knew it was something that I had to deal with. I had a very positive attitude until that moment. I felt like a piece of meat up on that table. It was as if I had lost control of my life and my body, and it was a very bad experience." Like

Anne McNamara, Barbara Bradfield, an earnest and intelligent woman, came to believe that the medical establishment could not be trusted to give her what she needed to beat her disease. She realized that she would have to become an activist and take charge of the decisions about her treatment.

"I tended to be very aggressive in my research," she says, "but a lot of women are like little sheep. They're led in to the doctor, they listen to what the doctor says, and that's what they do. And they don't look at anything else. And just from that first experience I had, I knew that I had to be in charge of things for myself. I couldn't rely on the doctor."

She found a new oncologist in Burbank. His first news was that she didn't have inflammatory breast cancer. "From that point on, I started getting all of my reports," she says. "I wanted everything in writing. I always knew what was going on." The doctor prescribed six months of chemotherapy to shrink the tumor, and then she underwent a mastectomy. She had more chemotherapy after the surgery, and then radiation.

Her treatment ended in the spring of 1991. "That's a scary time because while you're doing chemotherapy or radiation, you want to be done with it. But then when you're done with it, it's frightening not to be doing something to fight the cancer."

It was also about this time that Bradfield began keeping a journal, or a diary of sorts. She can't explain exactly why she chose to do this, but given the grueling rigors of her cancer treatment, it's likely she thought it would be therapeutic.

"I guess I just needed to write out my feelings," she admits. "It helped me out. I go back sometimes and read through and see what I've gotten over, what I've accomplished. Sometimes I'll read it and think, gosh, I've been scared and depressed a lot, but it really is like that's when I write is when I'm scared and depressed. I don't write all the good times in necessarily, and so I started trying to do that so I could have some balance when I go back and read it."

Like most other cancer patients, Bradfield began to investigate alternative therapies. Given the terrible odds—half of all cancer patients die from the disease—it is not surprising that so many seek help outside the orthodox regimens. Few pneumonia patients look for alternative treatments because the standard protocol is almost always successful. Gathering information, Bradfield attended a convention of practitioners and students of alternative cancer therapies in Pasadena, near her home, and began to consider which of the regimens—they ranged from vitamins, herbs, and other nutritional supplements to relaxation therapies, psychotherapy, hormone therapy, and homeopathy—to pursue. The convention made a strong impression on her. "I met people who were survivors. I met one lady who had had lymphoma and lesions on her lungs, and she was there seven, eight years later."

Suddenly, in November of 1991, Barbara Bradfield and her family faced a tragedy that made her cancer seem trivial. Driving home from a fitting for her prosthesis, Bradfield heard a radio report of a fatal accident at the freeway exit near her house. She thought nothing of the story and, when she got home, went ahead with preparations for the weekly Bible-study class that was meeting that night at her house. But soon members of her group showed up and broke the news that twenty-three-year-old Jennifer had died in the accident. She had been seven months pregnant with the Bradfields' first grandchild. The loss was indescribable. "We were real close. She was a real good support to me through all of the ups and downs of the first battle," says Bradfield. "She was in her seat belt," says Bradfield, recalling the terrible details of the tragedy. "We think—somebody behind her said that it looked like she had leaned over and then she overcorrected. And she was very sick all the way through her pregnancy. Either she got sick or she dropped something and leaned over to pick it up. One of the two. So I will never know, I guess, until I see her again. I plan to. There's nothing worse than losing your child. Nothing worse."

Nine months later, in August of 1992, she was sitting in one of her Bible-study classes, absently fingering the area around her neck. She felt a spongy, marshmallow-like growth. "You wonder how you could have something like that in you and not know. The minute I touched it, I knew what it was. I didn't hear much more of the Bible study that night." A needle biopsy confirmed that her breast cancer had recurred, and a CAT scan turned up a lesion on her lung. Bradfield had progressed to the "treatable but not curable" stage. The recurrence predicted in her original diagnosis had happened. Her doctor suggested she try high-dose chemotherapy, but she would have none of it. "Done with that," she says firmly. "If I'm going to die, I don't want to die bald and throwing up."

"I'm a realist," she says. "I read everything. When the cancer comes back in the lungs and in the lymph glands, then there's not a lot out here to give you hope for that situation. I had seen people who had gone through this chemo, chemo, chemo. They died anyway, but they died so sick. I felt that quality of life with my husband and kids was more important." Then the doctor, who happened to be a member of Slamon's loose network of Los Angeles–area oncologists, presented her with an option. "There's a guy doing a study at UCLA," he told her. "You want me to send your slides over?" Bradfield didn't pay much attention. "I said, 'I don't care. Go ahead. Sure.' And then I left."

She proceeded to investigate her options among alternative therapies. "I didn't feel like I was just opting to give up and die; I felt like I was choosing another method. Chemo hadn't worked for me the first time, so there was no reason for me to think it would work the second time around. I started researching all the clinics in Mexico. I figured my best bet was to detox and then to just work on making my body as strong as possible for as long as possible."

Returning to the Wellness Community in Pasadena for guidance, she decided to head down to Tijuana, Mexico, to check into a clinic that administers the Gerson program. Devised in the

1940s by a German-born physician named Max Gerson, it is billed as an effort to rid the body of poisons and summon natural healing mechanisms. Patients eat a low-fat, vegetarian diet and each day drink a dozen glasses of freshly pressed fruit and vegetable juices. The regimen also requires that the patient have a coffee enema six times a day to speed up the flushing out of the body's toxins. Like many other alternative cancer treatments, the Gerson program offers little hard evidence of its benefits, and the medical establishment has little use for it. But at that point, Barbara Bradfield held the medical establishment in low regard. She sank two thousand dollars into a special juicer and made a reservation to spend three weeks—at five thousand dollars a week—at the clinic. Just before she and Dean were to take off, she got the call from Dennis Slamon.

"He told me that he was doing this study and that my oncologist had sent him my slides and that he had tested them and I was one of the highest expressers of this gene—Her-2/neu—that he had seen," she says. He asked her if she would consider being part of his study. She wanted to know if the treatment involved chemotherapy. When he told her yes (his part of the phase I trial combined the antibody with cisplatin, which can cause harsh side effects, like nerve pain and damage), she turned him down and explained that she was on her way to the Gerson clinic. He said he respected her decision and thanked her for her time.

The next morning, he called her back. "He said, 'I've been thinking about this all night, and you just can't do this.' He said, 'What you have is too aggressive and will grow too fast for it to be treated with that kind of a regimen. You need something stronger than food.'" Dean urged her to hear Slamon out. She went to UCLA, where Slamon spent two hours describing the treatment to her. What impressed Bradfield more than the details of the treatment was Slamon's unbridled enthusiasm. "Dennis is very busy and very distracted sometimes, but at this point he was finally getting to test his treatment on human beings, and he was just so excited. Everyone there had this air of anticipation, all the nurses and everyone else who was involved." She agreed to join Slamon's first trial group for the humanized Her-2/neu antibody combined with cisplatin. The regimen would last three months to test the safety and dosage range of the Her-2/neu antibody in combination with cisplatin.

In that first group were fifteen patients. Some had gotten to Slamon the way Bradfield had, through the recommendation of their oncologists. Others had read about Diane Hinton in the *Los Angeles Times* or had otherwise heard about the treatment and had fought to get into the trial. All fifteen women would have been considered terminal. In seven, the breast cancer had spread to the bone; in others, to the liver, the lungs, or the brain. Bradfield's cancer had metastasized not just to her lymph nodes but to her lungs. At the start of the trial, she had sixteen lesions.

Phase I trials seldom yield information about a drug's effectiveness, but within weeks Slamon began to see positive results. Bradfield says the tumor that was visible on her neck made her a group favorite because everyone could actually see dramatic progress. Within two weeks, her neck tumor had shrunk by half. "Everybody else was so excited because they felt like they could see what was going on in me; therefore, something good had to be going on with them, too."

The group evolved into an extraordinarily close support system. Slamon had set up the sessions so that all the women were together in one big room. Says Bradfield, "I think all of us felt like this could be the magic bullet." "Everyone got attached," admits Slamon. "The nurses got attached to these women. The women got attached to the nurses. I mean, the one thing you don't do in oncology is get attached." The patients would come in with treats to share. "We would get real rowdy," says Bradfield. She got a particular kick out of a woman from Boston. "She was a very raucous kind of crass Jewish gal. She was hysterical. I just really liked her. She brought a cake from a porno cake place in Boston. It was this big cake with two big boobs in the middle. It said something funny about boobs and Dr. Slamon."

Several of the women were also exploring alternative therapies, and all shared whatever information they had. One woman of Chinese descent sought traditional remedies from China. "She'd bring back all these herbal things. She used to pass us out little packets with sea horses in them. They were awful. You're supposed to boil them. It was just disgusting," recalls Bradfield.

But the emotional attachment had its price. While the treatment showed some effect in some patients, it was hardly a cure-all for such desperately sick women. One young participant died almost immediately; her kidneys could not handle the treatment. Several others died over the next weeks, including the Chinese woman. Each death was a terrible blow for the group. "It was too hard when people started dying," says Bradfield. "We became very emotional."

Slamon and the other medical professionals were accustomed to deaths in phase I trials, where any positive effect of the drug is the exception. "To a person, these women said in group meetings that they were making a contribution even if the treatment didn't help them personally," Slamon says. "So you do feel bad when you lose patients. On the other hand, you've gained the knowledge that allows you to treat the next group of patients more intelligently." Still, the doctors decided that in future trials patients would be treated individually.

The standard measure of a positive response in a cancer trial is a reduction of the tumor mass by at least 50 percent. Based on that criterion, Bradfield's response was extraordinary. The tumor on her neck disappeared entirely, and scans revealed that she had between four and six lesions in her lungs, down from sixteen when the trial started. Slamon says that between 20 and 30 percent of his group had positive responses. Some, like Bradfield's, were dramatic, though no one had a complete elimination of the cancer. At the end of the three-month trial period, Slamon, in consultation with Genentech, decided that the drug combination worked well enough to extend the trial for at least some of the participants.

Looking for significant scientific results, not slightly effective therapy, Slamon and Genentech made some tough decisions. They chose to drop the seven women with bone metastases from the trial. Even though each said that her pain had subsided with the initial treatment, there was no way to follow their progress with objective measurements, such as CAT scans, so their cases would provide little additional information. "There was some anger," says Bradfield. "You know there's something out there that could help you, but you're not allowed to have it. It's very frustrating."

After the deaths and the exclusions, only Bradfield and four other women were permitted to continue with the experimental treatment. Before they could proceed, the five women had to wait while Slamon's team and Genentech submitted required paperwork to the FDA. Bradfield was excited about her progress and eager to move on to the next stage. "It was very frustrating because there was like a period of six weeks or more while they were getting organized. We didn't get back to the study right away. That was real scary 'cause you felt like it's going to grow again." At last, the five women began a second three-month cycle of antibody and cisplatin. One soon dropped out, however, because she could no longer tolerate the side effects of the cisplatin. Bradfield and the other three women completed the second course.

After the trial was over, Bradfield tried to stay in touch with the friends she had made. But over the coming months, husbands or other family members called her to say that her friends had died or were close to death. Beverly, the woman from Boston, was the last to succumb. "Bev's husband called me to say she was in and out of coma. And he put the phone up by her and had me talk to her," she says. "I had just gotten my tests at a year later saying I was clear. So he wanted me to tell her that. And Beverly, more than any of the rest of us, came into it saying, 'If this helps just one person, it's worth it.' "

Of the fifteen original volunteers for the Phase 1 study, only Bradfield survived. Repeated tests showed her to be totally cancer free. On each of many follow-up visits to Slamon, she asked what she should do next. Slamon had no precedent to follow. He remembers telling her, "We're where we haven't been before. We've used a new therapy and gotten a complete response with it. In someone who had sixteen to seventeen pulmonary nodules, do we continue the therapy? Do we stop the therapy? Do we stop the chemotherapy and continue the antibody? Do we stop everything together? There was no answer." One thing Slamon could not do was continue giving Bradfield cisplatin. The drug had already left her with nerve pain and hearing loss. More nerve damage would surely follow. So together they decided to try stopping it, Slamon remembers, "knowing that the tumor may come back or it may not."

Bradfield often reflects on why she was the one who survived. Some of her answers are medical. "I think, looking back, that I was stronger than most of them coming into it. I'd been off of chemo for a year and a half, and I had been eating well and taking good care of myself." Other answers are spiritual. "As a Jehovah's Witness, I believe that we get answers to prayers, and we can get guidance. And I believe very strongly that that's what I did, that I was guided to that study."

CHAPTER 7

The Mayor of
the Infusion Room

A t about the same time that Barbara Bradfield experienced her astonishing recovery in the phase I trials of Her-2/neu, Anne McNamara was nearing a turning point. She remembers a checkup she had with her oncologist in 1992. During the examination, he noted that she had been cancer free for five years, a milestone often used to categorize success or failure of cancer treatments. The five-year mark is popularly viewed as a sign that the patient has entered some sort of safety zone, that she is somehow less vulnerable to a recurrence. But for the individual patient, especially one with breast cancer, the milestone is virtually meaningless. Susan Love, who worked for Dennis Slamon when she was director of the Revlon/UCLA Women's Cancer Research Program, often told her patients, "When you die at ninety-five of a stroke, we'll know you beat breast cancer."

McNamara's case proved to be a cruel reminder of Love's wisdom. One year after that examination, she found another swollen lymph node and knew exactly what the problem was. When the doctor suggested another course of chemotherapy, McNamara responded, "We're not talking cure here, are we?" It was more a statement than a question.

The doctor urged her to consider an increasingly common option in cases like hers: high-dose chemotherapy with bone-marrow rescue, a procedure commonly known as a bone-marrow transplant and, more recently, a stem-cell transplant (although that phrase is misleading since the patient receives her own bone marrow). Knowing how physically depleting and dangerous the treatment can be, she rejected that option—at first. She began reading the medical literature and surfing the Internet, looking for new approaches to treat her cancer, anything but the high-dose treatment. That is how she found her way to an early trial of a vaccine designed to boost the body's immune system and thereby destroy any remaining breast-cancer cells.

McNamara's oncologist removed one of her swollen lymph nodes and sent it to a laboratory in California that was carrying out the trials. The approach was to grow large numbers of the cancer cells in culture, kill them with radiation, and inject the irradiated cells back into the patient as a vaccine. The hope was that this customized vaccine would prime the immune system to attack any live cancer cells remaining in the body. Ultimately, the idea failed to move beyond the initial testing phases. But McNamara never even got the chance to give the treatment a try. Six months after her oncologist sent off the lymph node, she got word that her cells would not grow in culture. While she waited, two more cancerous lymph nodes popped up. High-dose chemotherapy appeared to be her last resort. "I finally worked myself up to decide to do it," she says.

First employed in 1980, the high-dose regimen had become an increasingly common and ever more controversial treatment for advanced breast cancer. Some doctors hailed it as the most significant advance ever in treating metastatic breast cancer. Others saw it as an expensive, useless, and dangerous procedure that symbolized much that was wrong with American medicine. High-dose chemotherapy for breast cancer traces its roots to a similar treatment for a different cancer.

In the early 1950s, a Texan named Edward Donnall Thomas, a bearded, taciturn man, graduated from Harvard Medical School and then made his way to the University of Washington in Seattle, where he focused on leukemias and other cancers of the blood that had proved resistant to chemotherapy. His idea was to destroy a patient's bone marrow with radiation or chemotherapy and then replace it with marrow from a healthy donor. The concept is entirely logical. Leukemia is cancer of the bone marrow, the tissue that produces blood cells. Replacing the diseased marrow with healthy marrow should solve the problem.

But marrow donation turned out to be terribly difficult because the body often rejects donated marrow. Simultaneously, the donated marrow, which contains disease-fighting white blood cells, often attacks its new host. At first, Thomas succeeded only in transferring marrow between identical twins. But over decades, he discovered methods of matching donors, first close relatives and then even strangers. He developed drugs that would suppress the rejection response at least some of the time. But perfecting those treatments was painstaking for Thomas and his colleagues and even far more grueling and dangerous for the patients. Not only were the treatments themselves agonizingly painful, but in the interim between the destruction of the patient's bone marrow and the body's acceptance of the new marrow, the patient was highly vulnerable to almost any infection.

A physician who worked with Thomas recalled, "Of the first one hundred patients we wrote up in the first paper, only twelve survived. We put these people through hell, horrible pain and agony. It took a tremendous amount of chutzpah, arrogance, hubris—whatever you want to call it—to say we should continue and persist." But persistence paid off. Thomas eventually developed a transplant procedure that worked well enough for him to share a Nobel Prize in 1990. Thomas's research serves as a prime example of the ethos that often dominates experimental cancer treatment: yes, the treatment is poisonous, brutal, and often fails to work, but these patients would die anyway, and this is the best we have; if we persist, ignoring the cries that our treatment is inhumane, we can learn how to save more and more lives. That was certainly the attitude that often guided the development of high-dose chemotherapy for breast cancer.

In the late 1970s, researchers working with Thomas, who had moved across Seattle to the Fred Hutchinson Cancer Research Center, discovered that they could freeze bone marrow for indefinite periods of time and then defrost it and successfully transfuse it. Several oncologists then thought of a way to accomplish something they had wanted to do for a long time: elevate the dose of chemotherapy drugs. While the death rate for childhood leukemia and a few other rare cancers had fallen, oncologists remained frustrated by their inability to make much of a difference with solid tumors, the major killers. Certain kinds of cancers often responded to chemotherapy, which would bring patients maddeningly close to a cure, but all too often the cancer roared back with deadly consequences. Perhaps, they reasoned, the treatment would work more reliably if the dose were raised substantially.

The problem was that most of the major chemotherapy agents then available—such as 5-FU, Cytoxan, methotrexate, and Adriamycin—block DNA synthesis and kill dividing cells. Because bone marrow supplies the body with its enormous quantity of blood cells, bone-marrow cells divide rapidly. But if chemotherapy doses are too high, they demolish the bone marrow and kill the patient. That is where bone-marrow transplants come in. To raise the chemotherapy dose, doctors could remove a patient's bone marrow, freeze it, administer a whopping dose of chemotherapy—five to ten times what they could give when they had to worry about destroying the marrow—and then transplant the bone marrow after the chemotherapy drugs had washed out of the system. For this procedure, doctors need not bother with the dangers of tissue rejection because they are using the patient's own bone marrow in the transplant. Experiments with the procedure—known as ABMT, for autologous bone-marrow transplant—got under way at several medical-research centers. ABMT yielded some spectacular results with a few kinds of cancer, especially cancer of the lymph system. With little controversy, the treatment became the standard of care for some patients with lymphoma.

With breast cancer, the results were less successful. William Peters, a young faculty member at the Dana-Farber Cancer Institute, a Harvard Medical School teaching hospital in Boston, applied the procedure in 1980 and '81 to twenty-four women with highly advanced metastatic breast cancer, for whom chemotherapy had already failed to provide any further benefit. In three of them, the cancer disappeared entirely for a time. In six others, it regressed partially. In all nine women, the cancer returned in a matter of months, but the effect was strong enough to persuade Peters to concentrate on improving ABMTs for breast cancer.

Peters faced resistance from many quarters at Dana-Farber. "Many on the faculty said the treatment was brutal," Peters remembers. "The arguments even became sexist. They said women were too frail to withstand that much chemotherapy." The faculty committee that examines the ethics of experiments on humans was slow to approve the procedures. Craig Henderson, then head of Dana-Farber's breast service, objected to the experiments because, he said, there was an improper amount of basic science to back them up. "Dana-Farber was basically a small, conservative place," Peters says. So when Duke University, in Durham, North Carolina, offered him a position in 1984, he jumped at the opportunity. While Dana-Farber had fewer than fifty beds for all its cancer patients, Duke, eager to establish a national reputation for itself, gave Peters a sixteen-bed unit to be used solely for ABMTs for breast cancer. Those beds were almost always filled.

From the earliest cases, Peters, Karen Antman, who picked up the research at Dana-Farber after he left, and other oncologists using ABMTs said they were seeing women whose disease should have killed them live cancer free for months and then years. But these were assertions, not science. ABMTs for breast cancer were never proven to work unequivocally, as they had been for lymphomas. Some of the doctors doing bone-marrow transplants pointed out that 20 percent of women with metastatic breast cancer remained disease free for months or even years. But critics countered that these data did not come from trials comparing one treatment with another. They raised the possibility that doctors were subconsciously selecting women for the treatment who were more likely to do better. In a 1987 review of ABMTs for breast cancer, coauthor Antman concluded, "Whether high dose chemotherapy (with or without radiation) and autologous bone marrow transplantation are useful in the treatment of patients with breast cancer will have to be determined through an orderly progression of well designed studies." In other words, the treatment was experimental and unproved. "I had that sentence read back to me in court," Antman recalls.

ABMTs, in fact, became something of a legal lightning rod because the procedure is fantastically expensive, costing between one hundred thousand and three hundred thousand dollars. If a patient enters a trial for a new drug, the drug company always pays for the drug and often for part of the medical care. But patients or their insurance companies pay for clinical trials of new procedures, which are usually developed not by drug companies but by academic researchers. The insurance companies usually did not object to underwriting ABMTs when they were used for leukemia or lymphoma, which are relatively rare. But they balked at the idea of paying for the procedure as a treatment for breast cancer, a far more common disease. They were terrified at the prospect of covering tens of thousands of procedures that would cost them billions more dollars each year. The lines were drawn for one of the greatest legal battles in recent American medicine.

At first, doctors tried to circumvent the issue by denying that the treatment was experimental. Almost every health-insurance policy contains a provision prohibiting payment for experimental procedures. When the academic researchers tried to get the companies to pay for women to continue with what the researchers saw as more advanced trials, the companies refused. So leading researchers stopped describing the procedure as experimental. "We never used the *e* word," Peters says. They maintained that ABMTs were the best treatment available.

Under U.S. law, the FDA must approve a new drug before it can be used. But any doctor can perform any procedure if a hospital will allow it. Once the leading researchers stopped calling the procedure experimental, any hospital could have argued that attempts to limit the treatments to academic research centers represented restraint of trade. The sudden, widespread popularity of the technique was certainly due to many doctors' belief that it represented the best hope for their patients. But other doctors and hospitals undeniably regarded ABMT as a financial bonanza, playing right into the insurance companies' worst fears.

Insurers found themselves in a no-win situation. News reports regularly described the bake sales and church raffles organized to raise money for women who had been denied the "life saving" procedure by their health insurers. And patients, aided by their doctors, soon found a more effective way to get payment for the ABMTs: they went to court. In the typical case, one or more doctors testified that though the procedure may not work, it stood as the only hope for the woman to survive longer than a few more years. On the other side, doctors paid by the insurers testified that there was no proof that the treatment would do the woman any good and that it might kill her faster than the cancer. This scenario became so common that in the first years of ABMTs many of the mostly young, enthusiastic doctors who regularly performed the transplants spent a day or more every week in court trying to force insurance companies to pay for their prospective patients' treatment. The strategy often worked. Few judges or juries could look into the eyes of a patient, usually young and often a mother, and deny her a treatment that she and her doctors believed gave her her only chance at life.

By 1991, Blue Cross and Blue Shield was losing so many court cases that it offered to finance clinical trials to determine whether ABMTs work. The National Cancer Institute set up the trials, which were scheduled to conclude in 1993. Women would be randomly divided into two groups. One group would receive the ABMT and high-dose chemotherapy, and the other group would get the best standard chemotherapy. But the trials languished for years. Women told by their doctors that the procedure represented their last chance had no interest in joining a trial in which they might be assigned randomly to a control group. Eventually, the clinical trials did fill up, but as late as mid-1998 there were still no results.

As the ABMTs exploded in popularity, some physicians condemned their widespread use. Craig Henderson, who had moved from Dana-Farber to the University of California, San Francisco, derided some of his colleagues who "think they are performing miracles." He explains that "doctors with experience treating breast cancer know that a certain percentage of the patients with even the most seemingly hopeless forms of the disease will survive for many years with conventional therapy or even with no treatment. So when one or [a] few women do well, that doesn't prove that it is related to the specific therapy that was given. We simply do not have evidence that ABMT is much better than standard treatment. In fact, it may be shortening the lives of women who would have lived if they had not undergone the transplant."

Indeed, in the early days of ABMT, as many as 20 percent of patients died from the procedure itself—either in response to the massive doses of chemotherapy or as a result of an infection acquired during the time they had no bone marrow and thus no immune system. As doctors gained more experience with the procedure, the mortality rate fell below 5 percent, but when Anne McNamara decided the procedure was her best shot, it still sounded to her like a lot of risk for an unproved benefit.

By 1994, when McNamara opted for the high-dose chemotherapy, some insurance companies had decided to pay for the procedure. In December 1993, a California jury awarded $89.3 million to the family of a woman who died of breast cancer at age forty after Healthnet, her health-maintenance organization, had denied her payment for a high-dose chemotherapy treatment. Many insurers decided it was better to offer the service and try to negotiate lower rates with the hospitals than to continue to fight. McNamara had to switch insurance companies to get her treatment covered.

To prepare a patient for the high-dose regimen, doctors want to be certain the tumor will respond to the chemotherapy drugs. McNamara therefore went through two months of treatment with standard doses of 5-FU, Cytoxan, and Adriamycin. This was the first time she had taken Adriamycin in place of the less powerful methotrexate. Within a couple of weeks, she lost every hair on her body, an experience she calls "the most traumatic thing I have ever been through."

For many cancer patients, the loss of hair is devastating. Because it is such a visible and public sign that a person is sick and possibly suffering, hair loss is often a humiliating experience that can also produce feelings of shame. "I hated it, hated it, hated it," McNamara says with some vehemence. "I hated having to wear a wig. It started coming out about ten days after the first Adriamycin treatment. It took about a month before it was all gone. But it began to come out in patches, and it looked so horrible that I just cut it all off and put the wig on because I couldn't stand it." She detested wearing a wig but was grateful that the antinausea drugs kept the experience from being any more miserable. And when her swollen lymph nodes shrank, she was greatly encouraged.

After a three-week reprieve, she started treatment with Taxol, which doctors often give in tandem with the high-dose drugs. Taxol in its highest doses destroys not bone marrow but nerve cells. Two infusions three weeks apart left McNamara with shooting pains in her legs and lingering numbness in her fingers.

Before she could begin the high-dose chemotherapy, McNamara had to sign a consent form. Over the course of a dozen pages, it spelled out all the ways the treatment could backfire. "It went into great detail," explains McNamara, referring to the dreaded consent form. "All the things that could go wrong, and it was just awful. Your liver, we can't guarantee that your liver won't fail, and, you know, we can't guarantee that there won't be lung damage. Your kidneys might be permanently damaged. And on and on and on. And, finally, that we can't guarantee that when we give you back your stem cells, that they'll take. Well, to have it all spelled out. I knew this, all of these things were possible, but to see it spelled out. Like, gulp!" The document just about destroyed whatever confidence she had, but being the determined woman that she is, she signed it anyway.

By the time McNamara got the treatment, new technology was allowing doctors to remove stem cells, the progenitors of bone-marrow cells, from the blood. In 1989, doctors had found that they could bypass bone-marrow transplants by removing, storing, and replacing a relatively few stem cells. Once back in the bloodstream, the stem cells eventually produce billions of offspring, which repopulate the bone marrow. With stem-cell retrieval and other improvements, doctors had learned to reduce the length of the hospital stay.

The doctors gave McNamara a medium to high dose of Cytoxan and other drugs to kill her white blood cells and send a signal to her bone marrow to produce more stem cells. She spent a long night flat on her back in the hospital while a catheter circulated her blood through a machine that removes stem cells a few at a time. Then she got the high-dose chemotherapy over three days—Wednesday, Thursday, and Friday. She went home that weekend and suffered a high fever. The following Monday, she returned to the hospital to get her stem cells back and spent eight days in isolation, taking high doses of antibiotics and antiviral and antifungal medications while waiting for her white blood count to rise and her immune system to return to normal. For many women, the high-dose treatment is a horrendous experience. The enormous doses of poisonous drugs can bring on terrible physical pain and a variety of symptoms, as well as intense depression. In her marvelously dispassionate way, McNamara says, "It turned out not to be as bad as I had thought." She just hoped that this time she had been through the worst of it.

At about the time that McNamara was undergoing high-dose chemotherapy, Mary Bonesco seemed headed for the same treatment. In 1991, at age forty-seven, she had felt a few tiny lumps in her left breast. A specialist at a local hospital aspirated them with a needle and ordered a mammogram. With her results in hand, he told her that the lumps were nothing more than cysts and assured her that she was fine. Two years later, Bonesco noticed a second, larger lump in the same breast. At first, she did nothing. Caring for her mother, who had suffered a stroke, had left her desperate and emotionally drained. But the lump grew, and she could no longer ignore it. Her family doctor referred her to an acquaintance, the chief of breast surgery at Sloan Kettering. "But that's a cancer hospital," Bonesco remembers saying.

Like so many women stricken by the disease, Bonesco had never given breast cancer much thought. There was nothing unusual in her clean bill of health two years before the diagnosis of cancer.

The harsh truth is that no one knows what causes most cases of breast cancer. A few factors can slightly increase a woman's risk, including bearing a child late in life or not at all, drinking alcohol, or being overweight. But these are not major causes. In any case, Bonesco had her first child at age twenty, seldom drank, ate healthily, and kept herself fit.

Mary-Claire King, the renowned geneticist who first identified the gene BRCA1, which can lead to the rare form of inherited breast cancer, has studied the disease for more than twenty years. She says what strikes her most about the disease is "how extraordinarily healthy the women who develop breast cancer are. We are not talking about women who have done anything wrong. We are talking about women who have done everything right. And breast cancer comes along anyway." King notes that even the known risk factors are relatively insignificant. "There is no one thing we can put our finger on and say, 'That's the cause of breast cancer,'" she says.

Despite the debate about mammography and the public campaigns urging women to get the X-ray checkup, detection of breast cancer remains far less precise than many people imagine. Mammograms simply miss many tumors, and others may not be present at the time a mammogram is done but may grow so fast that they are unmistakable just a few months after the examination. At its best, mammography can locate a tumor as small as a pencil eraser. But by that time, the first rogue cell in the breast has divided, and each of its progeny has divided twenty times to yield a total of one hundred billion cells—all in that one small tumor. If the tumor cells are allowed to divide ten more times, the mass will weigh about two pounds and constitute a deadly malignancy. So the best a mammogram can do is locate a tumor two-thirds of the way along the route from initial cell division to certain cause of death. In January 1993, when Mary Bonesco first went to Sloan Kettering, her tumor had moved far down that road.

Her surgeon, Patrick Borgen, examined the tumor and arranged for her to have a needle biopsy as quickly as possible. What he found was a tumor so large that he did not believe he could remove it all. Under a microscope the cells looked closer in appearance to some primordial single-celled creature than to normal breast tissue, a sign of a highly malignant cancer. It all added up to a terrifying scenario. Borgen sat down with Bonesco and her husband, Vince, to detail his findings and describe her options.

"My whole world fell apart," Bonesco remembers. "All I was going for was a biopsy, and he's talking about mastectomy and bone-marrow transplants!" Borgen referred her to a young oncologist on the Sloan Kettering staff, a man with a well-established reputation in research circles. But like many other doctors, he could be self-important and condescending to his patients. Bonesco remembers her first visit with him: she was frightened and confused, and he had a bag packed, ready for an out-of-town trip. "He's telling me how serious my case was and what he planned to do. When I try to ask him a question, he says, 'Stop! Stop! Don't interrupt my train of thought! I'm in a hurry. Just listen.' " Bonesco was not about to stand for that kind of treatment. "That's when I really blew up, and I said, 'Your train of thought! What about my train of thought? What about me?' " She walked out and never saw that oncologist again.

Mary and Vince Bonesco's world is stable and loving, devoted to family and church. First-generation Americans, they have lived in the same house in a working-class Italian neighborhood in Brooklyn since shortly after they were married in 1966. Their first daughter was born one year later, and two more followed. When their youngest daughter started high school, Mary Bonesco began working at her church's day-care center. Every Thursday night, she and Vince serve meals at the parish's homeless center.

Both Mary and Vince stand about five foot eight and stay trim. She wears her black hair at shoulder length, and her easy smile emphasizes her high cheekbones. Even when discussing her illness, she never loses her warmth, leaning forward from time to time to touch a visitor on the arm as she speaks, her generosity of spirit always evident. Vince tends to be more serious. His shock of white hair tops a face weathered by a lifetime of outdoor work as a supervisor for Brooklyn Union, a local gas company. When they talk, they gaze at each other with obvious affection and often finish each other's sentences. It is impossible to visit in the Bonesco home and not get a sincere invitation to stay for dinner.

After her experience with the arrogant oncologist, Bonesco called Patrick Borgen. "I cannot deal with a doctor who speaks to me in that tone, in that manner," she told him. Borgen referred her to José Baselga, a then thirty-five-year-old from Barcelona studying in both the clinics and the laboratories of Sloan Kettering. Few practitioners of oncology radiate enthusiasm—a difficult attitude to muster in the face of so much suffering and death. But Baselga is almost joyful. "He is the kindest thing on earth," says Bonesco.

Bonesco was diagnosed with stage 3 cancer, meaning she had a large tumor with lymph-node involvement and a high probability of eventual metastases. Baselga wanted to try to shrink the tumor before surgery to give the surgeon a better shot at removing it all. He put Bonesco on high doses of Adriamycin, and she suffered all the usual side effects, including a low blood count and nausea. But the hair loss was the worst, an offense to the obvious pride she takes in her stylish appearance. Clumps of hair covered her pillow in the morning and clogged the shower drain until no hair remained on her head. She felt so ashamed that she never let anyone, not even Vince, see her without a scarf. Vince spent more than the family could afford to get her two of the best wigs he could find. She remembers with embarrassment her first day back at the day-care center. She wore one of her new wigs and hoped no one would notice. But as soon as she stepped out of her car, a parent shouted out, "Mrs. Bonesco! What'd you do to your hair? Why'd you change the color? Why'd you cut it? It looked so nice!" Bonesco recalls shouting back, "Mrs. O'Hara, leave me alone!" She rushed inside weeping and found a place to hide.

After three months on chemotherapy, Bonesco's tumor shrank enough for the surgeon to attempt removal. Given its size, a lumpectomy was out of the question. The surgeon performed a modified radical mastectomy, excising not just the breast but some chest and back muscle to try to get all the cancer.

Following standard procedure, he sent twenty-four of the lymph nodes that drain white blood cells from the breasts to the lab for analysis. When it spreads, cancer often begins by traveling through the lymph system. Generally, cancer in ten or more lymph nodes indicates a high probability of recurrence. The pathologist found cancer cells in sixteen of Bonesco's lymph nodes, yet another indication of a deadly cancer. Baselga considered the degree of lymph-node involvement and recommended that Mary go through high-dose chemotherapy, the same process that Anne McNamara had undergone, to forestall a recurrence. At the time, Sloan Kettering, following a research protocol, offered treatment only to women with metastatic breast cancer.

But Bonesco's cancer had not yet returned, although Baselga had little doubt that it would. He suggested that she look into the program at the University of Colorado Health Sciences Center in Denver, where Steven Jones had built himself a reputation as one of the nation's most aggressive practitioners of bone-marrow transplants. Jones operated several research protocols for high-dose treatment. They included many cases other doctors regarded as simply untreatable.

In April 1993, just two weeks after her mastectomy, Mary and Vince flew to Denver. "They took me on a tour of the hospital and said I'd be there for three or four weeks to kind of prepare me," says Bonesco. Then the hospital representatives hit the Bonescos with the news that the procedure would cost between $150,000 and $200,000, and as Vince remembers it, "They wanted the money up front." The Bonescos' health insurer, GHI, a division of Blue Cross and Blue Shield of New York, told them that it would not pay for the transplant.

Like many other doctors routinely performing high-dose chemotherapy, Jones had spent years helping his patients sue, or at least threaten to sue, their insurers for coverage. In fact, Jones pointed the Bonescos to a lawyer in New York City who had handled this kind of case before and had been victorious in the past against GHI. Dealing with the lawyer turned into an ordeal all its own. The lawyer started out by demanding a two-thousand-dollar retainer—a significant amount of money to a family whose finances were already stretched thin by expensive medical treatments. That retainer seemed to the Bonescos to cover nothing more than the lawyer's first few phone calls and letters to GHI. Before long, he was sending bills for more.

While Bonesco was back in New York awaiting the decision on the bone-marrow transplant, Baselga put her on another course of Adriamycin. She had already begun to suspect that things were not going well when she looked at the site of her mastectomy. "Here I am with this huge scar, cut up from one end to the other," she says, pointing from her sternum back to her shoulder blade, "and this thing was not healing."

A few nights after her first Adriamycin transfusion, she began suffering intense pain along the scar. Vince rushed her to Sloan Kettering, where Baselga confirmed her fears. "It was hard. It was red. It was not normal skin. It was not a normal reaction to surgery," he says, in his slightly accented voice. Biopsies on the scar confirmed his suspicions: the cancer had returned. Only three weeks after surgery, a new and virulent growth of cancer had already taken hold of the breast tissue that remained. Where Adriamycin had been effective in reducing the tumor just a few weeks earlier, it was now impotent. Bonesco's cancer had aggressively mutated to resist the chemotherapy.

Baselga offered Bonesco three choices: she could go through with the bone-marrow transplant at Sloan Kettering, where she now qualified for the procedure because her cancer had metastasized; she could try Taxol, then in its final trials; or she could join the phase II trial of the Her-2/neu antibody at Sloan Kettering. Baselga suspected that Mary would be a candidate for the antibody protocol because the virulence of her cancer was consistent with the behavior of tumors that overexpress Her-2/neu. And Baselga was in the ideal position to get Bonesco into the trial because Larry Norton had assigned the day-to-day administration of the trials to him. He explained to the Bonescos that the treatment was designed to counter the genetic changes that made Mary's cancer grow so ferociously and that the drug was still in the test phase, but earlier studies in animals and humans looked promising, and most interestingly, the drug seemed to have no side effects. He fully explained the other two choices as well, and left the decision up to Mary and Vince. "So I asked him point-blank, 'What would you do?' " says Bonesco. Baselga told her that Her-2/neu was at least worth a try. Taxol and bone-marrow transplant, he reasoned, would always be available to her if Her-2/neu failed.

The FDA protocol called for eleven weekly transfusions of the antibody. The trial protocol demanded that each case be documented with photographs. So every week, Bonesco had to pose for a hospital photographer with her mastectomy scar bared. It was utter humiliation. In the beginning, she says, "I would have tears running down, and José would be there putting a label on my chest and telling me which way to face." After several weeks, she stopped minding so much and even managed a joke or two about posing for *Playboy.*

Within three weeks, Bonesco began to see results when she examined her scar. "It started to heal," she says excitedly. "You could see that it was turning a pinkish color and that it was closing up. It was like a miracle happened." And all this without a single side effect. Baselga, who had been a believer in Her-2/neu, was still shocked at how quickly Bonesco responded to the treatment. He ordered biopsy after biopsy, and each turned up the same result: the large mass of cancer had simply disappeared. CAT scans, MRIs, and bone scans revealed no cancer anywhere else in Bonesco's body.

When the eleven-week protocol was coming to an end, Bonesco and Baselga faced a decision. Should she continue with the anti-body infusions and take the risk that if minute amounts of cancer still occupied her body, the disease might once again mutate to re-sist treatment? "We had a very emotionally difficult time because we had no idea how long this was going to work," says Baselga. They decided to take their chances and continue the therapy. Bonesco is still getting weekly infusions of Her-2/neu.

The nurses at Sloan Kettering all know Bonesco well, a welcom-ing, strong woman who fits the description of Earth Mother per-fectly. Most of the cancer patients pass through for weeks or months of treatment, and many return again and again as they bat-tle their disease. But Bonesco's weekly visits, now approaching six years, constitute a record, at least in the memory of the staff. Once hooked up to her intravenous drip, Bonesco often hangs the bag of liquid on a wheeled stand and tours the hospital, buying a few items at the gift shop or dropping in on hospitalized patients. Her parish priest appointed her his emissary and asked her to visit any of his parishioners hospitalized in Sloan Kettering. As she travels through the corridors, patients and doctors cannot help noticing that she lacks the appearance so typical of cancer patients—the pallor, the weakness, and the baldness. Bonesco knows this well. "They're all talking under their breath, asking, 'What is she doing here?' When I go in the hospital and I look at people [on chemotherapy], I think to myself, 'I used to be one of them, like Martians.' "

Bonesco was one of forty-three women with advanced cases of breast cancer in the phase II trials at Sloan Kettering and UCSF.

Just like Barbara Bradfield's phase I group at UCLA, the twenty-seven women at Sloan Kettering grew tight-knit. Although they were not all treated together, like Bradfield's group at UCLA, Bonesco managed to befriend just about every one of them, and with her easy charm and ebullience she soon became "the mayor of the infusion room." Over the years, other patients would seek her out for advice and comfort. Of the women in her original group, she knows that some of them got better, at least for a time, while others got no relief. "I would hear about this one passing on and that one passing on," she says sadly. "A lot of the time, the nurses would try to keep it from me, but I know that a lot of them didn't make it."

Other women went on to other therapies, and a few survived. The paper describing the phase II trial details the results of the initial eleven-week protocol period at Sloan Kettering and UCSF: In twenty-two of the forty-three women, the cancer continued to progress (patients were forced out of the study when their tumors grew). In fourteen women, the disease neither improved nor worsened. Eleven women saw some benefit, including one patient whose extensive liver metastases disappeared with treatment but ultimately returned and killed her a year later. And one woman enjoyed what doctors call in their understated way "a complete response." That was Bonesco, whose cancer went into total remission.

Given the nature of her disease and the unknowns still surrounding Her-2/neu, no one would go so far as to pronounce Bonesco cured. There's always the possibility that she could stop responding to the treatment. But Baselga is optimistic. "She had a lousy life expectancy," he says. "And she is doing great. Mary knows that without the antibody, she'd probably be dead."

The results of the Her-2/neu phase II trial would discourage any medical researcher except an oncologist. An antibiotic that cured one in forty-three infections would be deemed a failure. Certainly, the annals of cancer treatment are replete with stories of seemingly miraculous recoveries. But cancer experts regarded Her-2/neu with guarded optimism. For one thing, the results offered an important demonstration of the basic concept of antibody treatment. The Her-2/neu therapy had escaped the difficulties that had stymied antibody treatments for cancer in the past. The "humanized" antibody did not evoke an immune response, even with repeated doses. Nor did it make its target, the Her-2/neu protein, disappear. The old mantra that antibodies never work might have to be revised. The tumors shrank in one quarter of the women. But if one took into account tumors that either did not grow or shrank a little, more than half the women had positive responses, and this was in women with highly advanced breast cancer. The results raised an additional intriguing possibility. Because chemotherapy drugs are so toxic, doctors can administer them for only a finite amount of time. Then they must stand back and hope that the toxins knocked out the cancer so that it will not spread any more. But a nontoxic substance might be administered indefinitely, and even if it did not kill all the cancer, it might hold it at bay. Cancer cure had always been the great hope, but what if cancer control became an option?

The phase II trials at UCLA of the antibody with cisplatin produced results similar to those for the antibody alone. One in four women responded according to the strictest criteria, and one half experienced a benefit, even if temporarily. To be eligible for the study, Genentech required that a woman's cancer had to be spreading even while she took chemotherapy. The usual practice for clinical cancer trials in advanced patients is to accept someone whose cancer failed to respond sometime in the last six months. Slamon saw the requirement as yet more evidence of Genentech's ambivalence toward Her-2/neu. To fill all the slots, he had to ask his oncologist friends at other hospitals to help find patients. While none had the complete remission that both Mary Bonesco, in the phase II trial, and Barbara Bradfield, in the phase I trial, experienced, doctors saw powerful temporary remissions in women who were considered beyond any treatment.

Further trials would determine whether women with less virulent cancers could see more benefit, whether Mary Bonesco and Barbara Bradfield were just lucky or whether they were pioneers in a new era in breast-cancer treatment.

CHAPTER 8

Fighting for Compassion
and Access

M ary Bonesco was supremely lucky. She happened
to find a doctor who happened to be involved in
testing a drug for which she happened to qualify
and which happened to help her. But most women
in Bonesco's situation either don't hear about experimental treatments or can't get to them.

By 1994, promising news from the early trials at UCSF was
trickling out into the nascent community of breast-cancer activists
right in Genentech's backyard. They were learning the lessons of
the AIDS movement and were not prepared to take no for an answer. More and more women, some activists and some not, tried to
get access to the treatment, but Genentech resisted because supplies were tight and the company did not want to complicate the
already highly complex testing process. The lines were drawn for a
battle that would leave one of the most important legacies of the
Her-2 effort.

Bob Erwin and Marti Nelson never set out to be revolutionaries.
They were children of the South, politically conservative, obedi-
ent to the establishment, and never sought confrontation. Their life
together began conventionally enough. Marti, whose long dark

hair reflected her Lebanese ancestry, grew up in Baton Rouge, enrolled at Louisiana State University, and soon decided on a career
in medicine. In class, she met Bob Erwin, a slightly built, serious biology major from Tallahassee, Florida, who had always wanted to
start his own company. After college, Nelson continued on to LSU
Medical Center while Erwin went off to graduate school at the
University of Alabama, followed by training at Abbott Laboratories in Chicago and the University of California, Davis. But they
stayed in touch and saw each other over the summers when they
could.

When Nelson finished her residency in obstetrics and gynecol-
ogy at the University of Rochester, she joined Erwin in San Francisco, and they married in October 1986. They pooled all available
funds, mostly credit-card debt, so Erwin could start his company,
Biosource Technologies, which genetically engineered plants to
produce drugs. Nelson took a job with Kaiser Permanente, the
country's oldest, and one of its largest, health-maintenance organizations.

The next year, at age thirty-three, she discovered she had breast
cancer. "She had her first surgery on our first wedding anniversary," Erwin remembers. From the moment of her diagnosis, the
couple faced a series of decisions with no clear guidelines. Even
people as well informed as Erwin and Nelson found dealing with
breast cancer overwhelming. "Despite all of our scientific training
and her medical training, there are a lot of aspects of that disease
that one just doesn't really learn about until you absolutely have to
learn about it," he says. Nelson chose to undergo a modified radical mastectomy, standard treatment at the time. Knowing the dangers of recurrence and believing that medical progress was certain
to produce a more effective breast-cancer treatment one day, the
couple arranged to preserve a portion of her tumor in case it might
come in handy for any future treatments.

Nelson's doctors found no lymph-node involvement, so they would not have routinely offered her adjuvant chemotherapy. But Nelson and Erwin had read the studies that a year later led the National Cancer Institute to issue its emergency clinical alert urging that almost all breast-cancer patients get adjuvant treatment. They argued for chemotherapy, and both their surgeon and their oncologist agreed. Nelson went through a nine-cycle course of CMF—Cytoxan, methotrexate, and fluorouracil—that took almost a year but left her well enough to work until the final month of treatment, when she was just exhausted.

By mid-1990, Nelson was beginning to believe that maybe she had really put cancer behind her. Then, late that year, she found two new lumps. They had not appeared on a recent mammogram; they turned up during a self-exam. She had a second mastectomy, and this time she had six positive lymph nodes. She then went through four cycles of CAF: Cytoxan, Adriamycin, and 5-FU, a harsher treatment than CMF.

She had suffered hair loss and nausea three years earlier with CMF, but this time around the nausea was far worse. Erwin, close to developments in the pharmaceutical industry, knew of an extremely effective antinausea drug that had just concluded phase III trials and had been recommended for FDA approval: ondansetron, now on the market as Zofran. Nelson's oncologist hadn't heard about the drug, but after a long discussion of pros and cons, Nelson, Erwin, and the oncologist decided not to pursue it because it was not yet commercially available. "We did the easy thing," says Erwin. "That was the first time that we actually identified a drug that we knew would be helpful that we should get, [but] we made the decision not to push it." Nelson and Erwin were not yet ready to fight the system.

They went instead with the then standard nausea treatment, which did not help Nelson. "She just had a horrible time," says

Erwin. "We were basically still ... going with the conventional standard of care." Still, they closely followed scientific developments in breast cancer, reading the medical literature and attending conferences. Erwin says they soon realized that "what we thought was [the most] aggressive [treatment available] at the time wasn't getting translated into action that made a difference for her as an individual."

As Nelson practiced medicine and battled her own disease, the seeds of militancy began to take root in her outlook. She won a protracted battle with Kaiser Permanente management to set up what she called a code-pink system in its hospitals so women requiring an emergency cesarean section would get the prompt, adequate medical attention they needed. She tried to get the company to participate in more clinical trials of promising breast-cancer treatments.

Then, in 1993, her cancer reappeared, this time along her mastectomy scar. Her oncologist viewed it as an insignificant local recurrence best handled with radiation therapy. That recommendation confirmed Erwin and Nelson's skepticism about their doctors. They both knew that a recurrence after a mastectomy was a very serious matter. But they also knew no imaging technique available could have told them how serious the recurrence actually was. The radiation brought on pericarditis, an inflammation of the sac around the heart, which proved painful and debilitating. With steroids and other drugs, Nelson managed to keep the inflammation controlled well enough to be able to return to work.

But soon she started feeling aches and pains, particularly in her back. Her doctors first told her that the problem was probably due to her job; many gynecologists suffer back pain. A bone scan in the late spring of 1994 revealed no evidence of metastasis. By July, her pain had worsened, and she found a swollen lymph node in her neck. Erwin went to the hospital with her for a biopsy. He recalls that the pathologist performed the needle biopsy, examined it through the microscope right there, and told them that the results would take a day or two. "I knew as soon as he said that, that it was malignant. And I knew that *he* knew," says Erwin. "Five minutes later, the oncologist came in and said the pathology results were that it was malignant." Nelson's cancer had spread to her bones and liver. It was the first time that Erwin and Nelson felt truly betrayed by their doctors.

Almost from the beginning of Nelson's illness, she and Erwin had been involved in an activist group called Breast Cancer Action. BCA was founded in 1990 by Eleanor Pred, a lesbian activist in San Francisco who emerged as something of a star, appearing often on television and honored by *U.S. News & World Report* as one of the most notable women of 1991. She drew on the lessons of the women's health movement of the 1970s, which challenged a patriarchal medical profession dismissive of the concerns of women.

Before BCA came on the scene, almost all breast-cancer organizations focused on support rather than activism. Pred wanted an organization that would confront the establishment rather than spend its time in meetings where women consoled one another, dealing with their fears, pain, and grief. She followed the trail-blazing efforts of AIDS activists, many of whom were her close friends. Combining a mastery of medical complexities, slick public-relations skills, and often obnoxious confrontation, AIDS activists were forcing fundamental changes upon pharmaceutical companies, medical researchers, and the FDA. ACT-UP, the best known of the activist coalitions, remained a disparate group of people who argued endlessly about tactics and targets. But it made a huge difference. "They had tools and techniques that were very effective in dealing with corporate America," says Genentech medical director, John Curd, who was often the focus of ACT-UP's wrath.

A major goal of AIDS activists, especially in the days before effective combination therapy with protease inhibitors, was to gain access to experimental medications, whether they had been proved to work or not. The activists' rallying cry was "We are dying. We will test the drugs in our bodies." They sought to save one life at a time. If one could be saved, the philosophy argued, ten might be saved; if ten, a hundred, and so on. ACT-UP was part of a network of groups in San Francisco that disseminated information about AIDS treatments, including *AIDS Treatment News,* a respected activist newsletter that reported on all new therapies, from the most mainstream to the most wildly alternative. Over the years, Project Inform, a prominent activist organization based in San Francisco, offered not only information but also advice on smuggling drugs and at one time even carried out its own secret, illegal clinical trials.

One of the near-term goals of ACT-UP—pressuring drug companies to employ "compassionate access" that would give drugs to critically ill people before the drugs won FDA approval—was adopted wholesale by Pred and a few others. But such a confrontational approach was not a typical or natural one to take. As Nancy Evans, an activist in San Francisco and BCA vice president, puts it, "The breast-cancer community is largely uneducated on being political and making something happen. They haven't gotten beyond the pink ribbons and the racing for the cure."

One obstacle to whipping up furor in the breast-cancer community is that, unlike AIDS, the disease is often cured. Half of all women treated for breast cancer never need to be treated again, and many then prefer not to think about it. When women do require further treatment, they are often too sick and too scared to be politically active. But Eleanor Pred and the other San Francisco activists who joined with her wanted to follow the ACT-UP model and pressure pharmaceutical companies for access to unapproved drugs. Like AIDS activists, breast-cancer activists fought for positions on government committees that influence their fate, including the FDA and National Cancer Institute committees in Washington. After Pred died of her disease in October 1991, ACT-UP and BCA joined in a demonstration in her memory outside the Japanese consulate in San Francisco. Daiichi Pharmaceutical Corporation of Tokyo had developed a drug called SP-PG that might have been useful for both breast cancer and the AIDS-related cancer Kaposi's sarcoma, and the activists demanded it immediately. Daiichi did not acquiesce. The drug ultimately proved ineffective.

Gracia Buffleben and her husband, George, took Pred's place as the link between BCA and ACT-UP/Golden Gate. The conservative-looking, middle-aged couple certainly stood out among the tattooed and body-pierced ACT-UP crowd. A dynamo of a woman, Buffleben was a mother of three who had been a Girl Scout leader in Dublin, a small, working-class town in the far eastern reaches of the San Francisco Bay area. She had been diagnosed with breast cancer in 1987, at age forty-two, and when her disease spread to her lungs and bones in 1992, she gave up her nursing career to devote herself full-time to fighting the medical establishment that she believed had let down so many women.

Soon after she joined BCA, in one of the arcane factional battles so common in activist organizations, Buffleben left the group to form the Breast Cancer Treatment Issues Committee of ACT-UP/Golden Gate. In one of her first victories, she persuaded the pharmaceutical giant Burroughs Wellcome to adopt a compassionate-access program to distribute a new anticancer drug, called Navelbine, similar to Adriamycin, to five hundred women with breast cancer.

The activists at BCA and ACT-UP were hearing about the trials for Genentech's extraordinary breast-cancer treatment. UCSF was then participating in the Specialized Program of Research Excellence, or SPORE, sponsored by the National Cancer Institute. SPORE's goal was to get researchers and physicians from various disciplines to talk to each other. At first, the SPORE meetings excluded all but professionals, but in response to activist pressure Craig Henderson, the new chief of oncology at UCSF, agreed to admit patient representatives. Marti Nelson and Bob Erwin volunteered to attend in 1992.

Erwin remembers the atmosphere of suspicion as the first meeting opened. "Some of these researchers had been funded by NCI and other government agencies for years to build careers around breast cancer, [yet] many of them had never met a patient with breast cancer before. Some of them had never even talked to a doctor who treated breast-cancer patients!" Nevertheless, it was not long before the researchers and the activists viewed each other with mutual respect. Discussion at the SPORE meeting eventually came around to Her-2/neu and the phase II trials then in progress at UCSF, Sloan Kettering, and UCLA. The optimistic results shed a bright ray of hope for both the researchers and the patients.

Gracia Buffleben and her impassioned allies soon decided to make compassionate access to the Her-2/neu antibody a major priority. Not only did it appear to be a possibly effective nontoxic treatment, but Genentech manufactured it right in ACT-UP/ Golden Gate's backyard. What better target could they ask for? Buffleben got a call from one woman who had participated in the phase II trial at UCLA and had been dropped when her cancer progressed; the caller knew that her disease had gotten worse, but she still believed that the treatment had helped slow the disease's progress. Word on Her-2/neu had also spread on the infusion-room circuit. "You know when you get chemo, you go into this infusion room. It's like a beauty-parlor chair. Women talk," explains Marilyn McGregor, a veteran of BCA and ACT-UP and a ferocious fighter. "They were doing the phase II at UCSF here in San Francisco. And so some of the participants noticed when one of them started looking pretty good. And so people began to hear about Her-2 through the grapevine."

The experience of Marilee Bronson, a BCA member and phase II patient at UCSF, made demands for Her-2/neu especially compelling. Bronson was suffering from recurrent metastatic breast cancer and did not want to go through another round of chemotherapy. She had heard about the Her-2/neu trials and fit the protocol. After her round of treatment in the trial, she lived eighteen more months. "She came back like a phoenix from the ashes," says Marilyn McGregor. "So we thought, 'This is serious. This woman got almost two years of life that she wouldn't otherwise have had.' So we thought, 'We need to work with Genentech so that other women can get this drug even though it's not approved and even though they don't fit the protocol.' "

Gracia Buffleben managed to get tested early on. Even though she could not benefit from the Her-2/neu antibody, she made it one of her top priorities. Ever flamboyant and often appearing bald from the chemotherapy at meetings, she spent much of 1994 trying to get in touch with decision makers at Genentech, where researchers were designing the pivotal phase III trials, the final stage of testing that would determine whether Her-2/neu would come to market. Following the ACT-UP model of direct negotiation, her strategy was to meet with the principal investigator, Tom Twaddell, and the head of clinical trials, John Curd, to get a copy of the protocol. She hoped the activist community could be given a chance to suggest alterations in the protocol—like opening the trial to a wider group of patients. AIDS activists had persuaded companies to make similar changes in trials for AIDS drugs. Genentech tried its best to ignore her but finally did grant her a pro forma meeting. "It was with the security person or the PR person," says McGregor. "Very low level. Kind of patronizing."

In fact, Genentech had no interest in giving out the unproved drug to a few dying women. As John Curd puts it, "Genentech's policy at that time—and it wasn't a written policy, but it was as close to it as you could have—is, We do not provide single-use, compassionate-use programs." From the company's viewpoint, this made eminent sense. Giving an experimental drug to a few people before it was proved effective wasted resources, time, and money that should be spent on either proving whether this drug works or searching for other drugs that might.

Ever since Marti Nelson's cancer had recurred in 1993, she and Bob Erwin suspected that she might benefit from Her-2/neu because her disease—aggressive and striking at a young age—fit the profile of a Her-2/neu overexpresser. They thought they might be able to obtain the antibody under a compassionate-use program, but they remained leery of rocking the boat. Retiring by nature, they were not eager to enter the fray.

But as excitement over the treatment stirred in the activist community, Erwin and Nelson faced their own hurdles with the medical establishment and Genentech. The first thing they had to do was establish that Nelson was positive for the gene, which meant getting a sample of her tumor tested. "That's when the real bureaucratic runaround started," says Erwin. "The most amazing and frustrating aspect of this thing was that we couldn't even get the assay [the genetic test] done." They needed to get the specimen sent from the Kaiser Permanente hospital where she was treated to UCSF, which could either test it or send it to Genentech for testing. "For some reason, different people [would] say, 'Well, it's not us; it's them.' Or, 'The committee is reviewing.' Or, 'It takes time.' Or whatever."

A historic distrust between the Kaiser Permanente system and UCSF was one of the problems. When the industrialist Henry Kaiser set up the country's first HMO after the Second World War, many doctors regarded his system of prepaid health care for his workers as an evil experiment in socialized medicine, especially when it opened its doors to community enrollment. It was so reviled that the local chapter of the American Medical Association refused membership to Kaiser doctors. UCSF remained the bastion of traditional fee-for-service medicine. By the early 1990s, both institutions were fighting for patients in the face of challenges from corporate-run HMOs, which could cut medical costs far more deeply. But a gulf still separated Kaiser and UCSF.

Debu Tripathey, who was overseeing the Her-2/neu trials at UCSF, blamed the delay on the realities of managed care, which has stripped medical staffs to the very minimum. "This is something we're encountering a lot," he says. "Across the country, the departments like radiology, pathology, laboratory medicine, have all had severe cutbacks in their funding. They've had to lay off a lot of personnel, so when a request comes in out of the blue [to] go out, [to] go to the archives and [find the tumor sample], that... takes literally an hour of one person's time to go out and get it, and then the pathologist has to make sure the block contains tumor, so he's got to make some slides and look at them. It ends up being quite a time sink; in the past, pathology departments had no problem with it 'cause they had plenty of people running around who could do this."

A simple bureaucratic roadblock may have stood between Marti Nelson and the test, but Marilyn McGregor, always outspoken, sees it differently. "It was a combination of Kaiser's incompetence, UCSF's incompetence, Genentech's incompetence, and nobody really caring to have her tumor tested." Erwin believes that something more insidious was going on. "Nobody was giving us the straight story. Everybody was blaming somebody else. What we eventually figured out was that one way or the other Genentech was blocking it because they did not want women to find out if they were eligible for the study and then not be able to put them on the trial." The refusal was amazing because Marti Nelson was a physician who knew the UCSF doctors from the SPORE meetings and had even consulted them for second opinions on her own patients.

As Erwin and Nelson were trying to get access to Her-2/neu, Nelson's cancer was spreading. Her doctor tried Taxol, to no avail. Infusions of 5-FU were ineffective. She was desperate. Gracia Buffleben decided to use Nelson's story to force Genentech to pay attention. At first, Nelson and Erwin resisted, but Buffleben was ready to make whatever trouble needed to be made.

"Gracia had been talking to UCSF and talking to Genentech and helping a lot on our behalf because, even in the fall of ninety-four, when we knew she was dying, we were still too much a part of the establishment," says Erwin. "In the early stages, Marti didn't want to alienate people and make them uncomfortable. She viewed herself as a professional member of the medical community, which she was. And I run a biotech company. I have a professional position in the community of biotech people." He saw himself on the same side as Genentech.

For Erwin, a mild-mannered man, the turning point came in mid-October 1994. "One day Gracia called me and Marti. By then Marti was really sick. She was on oxygen and finally had had to stop all of her work and was confined to bed and made only short trips out of the house. We were reviewing the latest frustrations in not being able to get the Her-2 tests run. And [Gracia] said, 'You know, this isn't just a philosophical point or an abstract issue that we're dealing with. This is Marti's life.' I realized this isn't statistics. This isn't an experiment. This is one person, and either she lives or she dies. There's no gray area. The decisions we make right now are going to influence whether she lives or dies. Who cares what people think?" And Nelson agreed. "She by then really knew she was being lied to," says Erwin. "Finally, she said, 'It doesn't matter to me. Tell them to do whatever they want to do, and I'll help however I can.'" Buffleben, big, bombastic, and larger than life, had done her job well: by convincing this normally reticent, nonconfrontational couple that they were looking at a question of life and death, she had at last succeeded in persuading them to become activists.

Nine days later, Nelson finally learned that she had tested positive for Her-2/neu. Buffleben, working with ACT-UP/Golden

Gate, organized a fax and phone zap, one of ACT-UP's favorite weapons. From phone books and sympathetic informants inside a company, the activists learn the direct phone and fax numbers of anyone in the company who might make a difference; then they clog up those lines in an attempt to paralyze the company. The fax and phone zap struck Genentech on November 8, 1994. The next day, Marti Nelson died. She was forty.

In Nelson's honor, Buffleben decided to organize a protest and began planning it at her funeral. "Gracia comes up to me in her most conspiratorial mode," says Marilyn McGregor, "and whispers, 'I have a great plan. We're going to drive up on the lawns of Genentech. Do you want to join?' So I said, 'Count me in.'" Breast Cancer Action chose not to be an official sponsor of the protest because, as Nancy Evans explains, "people on the board were worried about (a) being arrested, (b) getting their cars towed, (c) having to pay fines." Some members worried that they might some day need the drug and did not want to alienate Genentech (one board member did, in fact, end up getting Her-2/neu).

About forty breast-cancer and gay activists descended on Genentech's South San Francisco campus in a fifteen-car "funeral procession" on December 5. The demonstrators were a disorganized lot. At Genentech, there is no identifiable central headquarters, no obvious target for a demonstration. But the protesters, some holding posters of an angelic-looking Marti Nelson in her chemotherapy turban two weeks before her death, still managed to block roads and otherwise make a nuisance of themselves, honking horns and blaring sirens. "We did these circles of the various campus buildings and then parked the cars where it says 'No Parking.' And then we drove up on the lawns. We had a couple of really loud screamers from ACT-UP or other places," recalls McGregor. Gracia Buffleben drove her car up on a lawn and handcuffed herself to the steering wheel.

Many of the demonstrators were disappointed that they failed to attract much outside attention. McGregor, who handled the public relations for the event, says that they would have gotten more news coverage if robbers had not struck a downtown San Francisco bank at precisely the same time. But inside Genentech, the demonstrators accomplished far more than they could know. "It made vice presidents and senior vice presidents aware that the activist community could come on-site," says John Curd. "That demonstration made a statement to the people at the top level of the company that you are vulnerable to this kind of thing and unless you are willing to deal with this issue, they are going to escalate the conflict in ways you don't like."

The company could only take so much harassment and eventually sent out a representative to try to sound a sympathetic note and calm the protesters. According to McGregor, "Some guy came out and said, 'I'm a scientist working on the AIDS cure. Why are you here? You're making too much noise.'"

Meanwhile, the nondemonstrating members of BCA had asked Genentech to meet with them that afternoon, and the company agreed. The meeting proved far from satisfactory for either side. McGregor said the Genentech representatives "were just in there saying, 'Let me tell you girls about how a clinical trial works.' They gave us a slide show," she remembers. She and the other activists walked out after twenty minutes, fed up with what they saw as Genentech's patronizing attitude. Barry Sherman, who was then vice president for clinical research, also walked out, because the women would not accept what he thought were profoundly logical reasons for refusing compassionate access.

This angry failure to communicate disturbed John Curd, who was supposed to be running the meeting. Curd, who then headed Genentech's Immunology and Oncology Division, saw himself trapped in the middle of a dispute that could cost him his job. He was struck by a sense of déjà vu: Genentech had tried to develop several products that researchers hoped would prevent or treat infections in AIDS patients. The efforts failed, but they attracted the attention of the local ACT-UP chapter, which made demands for compassionate access and attempted to change the trial design. ACT-UP never seemed to get satisfaction from Genentech. But the activists had won John Curd's respect: "They're a tough group. Their activism was not misguided." Curd realized that while only a few patients were demanding compassionate access to the Her-2/neu antibody, they could bring the company big trouble.

Genentech's senior management sought the help of several female employees, including scientists. It also turned to its Washington office. In 1977, soon after the company opened its doors, Congress was considering laws to restrict genetic engineering. Genentech founders Herb Boyer and Bob Swanson went to Capitol Hill to persuade lawmakers to kill the proposed legislation. The company put a lot of stock in its Washington operations from then on. Now, to deal with ACT-UP/Golden Gate and BCA, Genentech's full-time Washington lobbyist, Walter Moore, put the company in touch with national breast-cancer activists. "I wanted to have support from a high level of a representative body of women with breast cancer if this thing got out of hand," Curd says. Moore hired the lobbying firm of Bass and Howes, specialists in women's health issues, which arranged for Genentech officials to fly to Washington to meet with Frances Visco, chairwoman of the National Breast Cancer Coalition.

Like Marilyn McGregor, Eleanor Pred, Gracia Buffleben, and Nancy Evans, Visco propelled herself into activism after her own diagnosis of breast cancer, at age thirty-nine in 1987. She, too, was appalled that breast-cancer organizations spent most of their energy in self-help groups rather than trying to change a system that she believed ignored the needs of women with the disease. She joined a local group in Philadelphia and attended the first summit meeting of local breast-cancer organizations in Washington in

1991. Visco, whose warm smile can disguise the tenacity that earned her a reputation as a prominent Philadelphia litigator, says her first national activists' meeting was "like this epiphany. I walked in, and I said, 'This is where I need to be. This is where my soul is, my heart is.' And I got involved from the very beginning."

Visco quit her law firm to devote her life to the politics of breast cancer. While the San Francisco activists met in each other's homes and spoke of fax zaps and similar guerrilla tactics, Visco moved into a world of one-thousand-dollar-a-plate corporate-sponsored black-tie dinners and testimony before key congressional committees. Under her leadership the coalition achieved a resounding success in its first year, winning a $43 million (50 percent) increase in federal spending on breast cancer. The following year, 1992, the coalition demanded and got an astonishing increase of $300 million under a new program for breast-cancer research it engineered in the Department of Defense.

Like the San Francisco women, Visco believed that she and others trying to effect political change for breast cancer owed a debt to AIDS activists. "We saw what they could do when they brought their voice to the political process. And we said we need to do that for breast cancer." But Visco did not believe it was necessary to superimpose the ACT-UP model of confrontation on breast-cancer activism. AIDS activists, she said, had to overcome enormous prejudice to get scientists and the public to pay attention to their plight. "There is no one who would tell you that they don't want to pay attention to breast cancer," Visco says. "The issue really is, What do they want to do about it?"

Visco has little use for the goal of trying to save one life at a time. What she wants are clinical trials—lots of them—to find better treatments. "How else are we ever going to find out what works? We have no cure. And we have these horribly toxic therapies that are of minimal effect in breast cancer. And we don't even know which women benefit from the incredibly toxic therapies that we give all women who present in a certain way.

"I would love to see a time when a woman goes to her oncologist and she is given a therapy that we know works, and not therapies that the doctor hopes will work or believes might work because it worked in another disease or it worked for two other patients that he treated." Visco considers clinical trials to be the only path to that goal. And she believes that doctors, the government, drug companies, and above all, patients need to understand that.

If the Genentech representatives thought that Visco would provide them an escape from the pressure applied by ACT-UP/Golden Gate and Breast Cancer Action, they misread her. She told Genentech in no uncertain terms that the company had no choice. John Curd remembers, "Fran Visco said to me, 'John, I agree with you intellectually and scientifically. Compassionate use does not make a lot of sense. I'd like to see the data. But this is not an intellectual issue. This is an emotional and political issue. And politically, you have to have a compassionate-use program.'"

Early in the meeting, Visco presented the Genentech representative with an ultimatum: "There is going to be an access program, or the meeting is over." She told Genentech she wanted a role in designing the upcoming phase III trials and her organization wanted representatives on the committee that planned the experiment as well as on the Data Safety and Monitoring Board. She believed that Genentech "wanted us to bless whatever compassionate-use policy" it decided on. But she demanded that her group help design it and refused to exclude ACT-UP from the negotiations.

In April 1995, Genentech invited both Visco and Marilyn McGregor of ACT-UP/Golden Gate to a meeting of physicians who were helping to design phase III trials. The so-called investigators' meeting took place in Reston, Virginia, outside Washington, D.C. The two women took an instant dislike to each other, fueled in

large measure by McGregor's realization that Genentech was trying to use Visco to neutralize her own organization's power. After
her discussion with Visco about the difference in the availability of
drugs for AIDS and for breast cancer, McGregor, a social worker
who had spent most of her career working with ghetto addicts, says
the corporate lawyer showed an ignorance of the key issues. Visco
complains that ACT-UP wanted expanded access, but "they really
didn't have a specific policy." Neither woman's view of the other
was fair or accurate, but they would remain adversaries on the same
side of the issue. Eventually, each woman presented her organization's separate demands: BCA and ACT-UP emphasized compassionate access; all the activists, including NBCC, wanted a role in
designing the phase III trials. They waited for the company's response.

Following the December 1994 demonstration, and even before it
lobbied Fran Visco, Genentech began meeting with the San Francisco activists. In January 1995, the company shared some of its
plans for the phase III trial and solicited the activists' comments.
By then, Gracia Buffleben's condition had so deteriorated that she
could not take part; Marilyn McGregor headed a committee rep-
resenting the activists. Among its members were Ricki Dienst and
her husband, Bob Moulton. Dienst, like Marti Nelson before her,
would soon prove a formidable symbol in the fight for compassionate access to Her-2/neu.

A clinical psychologist from Berkeley and part-time faculty
member at UCSF, Dienst was diagnosed with breast cancer in
1986 and was very active in the San Francisco cancer-support
community. In mid-1994, she had tried to get into the Her-2/neu
trials. Although she knew she was Her-2/neu positive, she was ineligible for the protocol, supposedly because she had already had
too much chemotherapy, although she had trouble nailing down a
precise answer. Like Marti Nelson, she was stymied by some combination of confusion, incompetence, and bureaucracy. In the

spring of 1995, she taped a message for her fellow activists. It reveals the voice of a woman who knows her death is near and can barely contain her anger at her inability to get a drug she believes might save her life. "My personal energy is increasingly diminished, and my disease has progressed significantly since I began trying to gain access to Her-2/neu, which is over at least six months now, maybe a little bit longer, and unfortunately, I guess, at the current rate that progress is being made on all of this, it is probably quite likely that I am going to die before I actually gain access to this treatment. But I'm still pursuing it because I think there are larger issues that need to be faced about this, and maybe my case and my pursuit of my case will help others, if not myself, although it isn't entirely altruistic—I do want to help myself, of course."

When Dienst got word that she could not join the trial, she took her case to Debu Tripathey, the oncologist overseeing the trial at UCSF. He tried to intervene with Genentech, but the company remained adamant about needing a very homogeneous test group in phase II so that it could measure the results as accurately as possible.

Tripathey describes Genentech's dilemma: "If you start making exceptions and deviating from your protocol, then you get a lot of patients whose results are not going to help you understand whether a drug works or not. All you're doing is delaying our ultimate knowledge of the drug's efficacy and being able to get it out to the public." Still Tripathey refused to accept that argument fully, believing, as the activists did, that the company could give the drug out compassionately, follow the women who got it, and still "get clinically meaningful data out of it that will contribute to getting the drug approved."

Tripathey phoned John Curd to try to get the drug for Dienst. Curd refused. Dienst's own oncologist, Jeffrey Wolfe at UCSF, put in several calls to Curd. "On July 15," recalls Bob Moulton, "we had an appointment with Wolfe, and it was at that meeting that he spoke to

Curd for quite a long time, urging him, asking him. Curd said no, and Wolfe was convinced they were going to stonewall. I saw Ricki kind of—for the first time—crumble. I mean, she was very tough and had been fighting nine years. I thought, 'My God, she's given up.' It was a very hard moment."

But Curd's denials further radicalized Dienst and turned her into an even higher-profile cause for the compassionate-access movement. "It had become a political issue," says McGregor. "What may have passed unnoticed in the past they couldn't do at this point because everyone knew Ricki." And even though she was getting weaker by the day, she was ready to make trouble. McGregor organized another fax zap of Genentech, and Dienst got a doctor to write a public letter to the company, arguing her case. Tripathey had to recuse himself since he was working with Genentech on the trial, so Dienst's bone-marrow-transplant doctor wrote the letter. Bob Erwin, recovering from the death of his wife, took it upon himself to do a one-man fax-phone zap on Roche, which owned a sizable chunk of Genentech.

A few days into the zap, Dienst got a call from John Curd, who tried to explain Genentech's position. He ran through the by-now familiar litany: the treatment was prohibitively expensive and in very short supply. Moulton says Curd even told Dienst that "if we give the drug to you, some other woman won't get it." But Moulton believes that "it really boiled down to money." Genentech just wanted Dienst to go away. "They had a real, especially intense need to get her quieted down," he says. "If they gave it to anyone, especially someone with a relatively high profile like her, it would have been very hard to avoid a compassionate-usage program, and they just didn't want to do that."

Curd says denying the drug to Dienst and others caused no great difficulty. "I was a practicing doc. I had taken care of hundreds, probably thousands of people who have died from bad diseases. I have no trouble personally engaging people with bad diseases. But I also know that our job here at Genentech is to develop and test therapies that might make a difference."

Ricki Dienst died on August 1, 1995. BCA and ACT-UP/Golden Gate took her story to the press and this time got noticed—at least in the alternative papers. One particularly damaging article appeared in the August 16 issue of the *San Francisco Weekly* under the headline AS THEY LAY DYING: BREAST CANCER ACTIVISTS RAGE AT GENENTECH FOR WITHHOLDING AN EXPERIMENTAL DRUG. It set out the details of Marti Nelson's and Ricki Dienst's losing battles with the company. Once the darling of San Francisco for its pioneering role in the biotechnology industry, Genentech was now being portrayed as heartless and, through its actions, a contributor to the deaths of two women.

By the time of the article (which contained many inaccuracies), Genentech had already decided to implement a compassionate-access policy and was working out the final details, a situation the company tried not to publicize for fear of setting off a flood of requests that it could not yet handle. So with the compassionate-access program quietly in development as public outrage over Marti Nelson's and Ricki Dienst's deaths mounted, the company teetered on the edge of a public-relations free fall. Soon after the demonstration in December 1994, Laura Leber, the company's twenty-eight-year-old director of corporate communications, joined the task force to find a solution to the problem of expanded access. It was Leber's job to tell reporters and individual patients why the company was refusing to give out the drug in a compassionate-access program. At the outset, there appeared to be no logic in the denials. She detested the role, and within the company she was one of the strongest voices in favor of implementing a program. "If my company gave me a directive and I could see the logic in it, I would support it," she says. Working with Fran Visco's group and with the

Bay-area activists, she helped hammer out the details. Two days after Ricki Dienst's death, Leber issued a Genentech press release announcing an expanded-access policy. The Bay-area activists had achieved their goal.

One problem Genentech faced was short supplies of the drug. The company had encountered unexpected technical problems scaling up production from the amounts needed for the phase II trial to the much larger amounts necessary for phase III. At this point, Bob Erwin played a crucial role as a go-between. Just before his wife died, he had set up the Marti Nelson Cancer Research Foundation, dedicated to securing experimental treatments for dying cancer patients. At first, Genentech resisted working with him, fearing he might still be angry about his wife's failure to get the drug. But Erwin, a soft-spoken man, suppressed whatever anger he still felt. The Genentech executives soon found that besides being an activist, Erwin was a biotechnology executive himself, spoke their language, and shared many of their values. After signing a confidentiality agreement, Erwin certified for the activists that Genentech could produce only enough of the drug for twenty-five patients in the expanded-access program each quarter.

To allocate the drug, the company adopted the idea of a lottery, run by an outside, private company. Physicians with patients who had failed other forms of treatment but who had tested Her-2/neu positive would submit their names, which were then chosen at random by the outside company. Every woman who got the drug would have to be treated under the auspices of a hospital as part of an experimental program. About a dozen hospitals across the country offered the drug to women who "won" the lottery. The formal experimentation guaranteed that Genentech would get data on each woman in exchange for the drug. The lottery system avoided any appearance of favoritism toward friends of Genentech employees, activists, or anyone else. As news reports over the next few years described how women were dying because they had lost in the lottery, Laura Leber could say with a clear conscience that the system was fair.

Marilyn McGregor, Nancy Evans, Bob Erwin, and the other San Francisco activists could point with pride to more than three hundred women who got the drug through the expanded-access program before it won FDA approval. In fact, the expanded-access program, which Genentech had resisted so strenuously, produced data that ultimately would help the drug win FDA approval. As time passed, Genentech grew more comfortable with the San Francisco activists. In addition, its relationship with Fran Visco and the National Breast Cancer Coalition, forged as a defensive response to those same activists, would prove beneficial to Genentech for testing and marketing the new drug.

Fran Visco's organization managed to appoint one of its officers, Kay Dickerson, a breast-cancer survivor and an epidemiologist at the University of Maryland, to the critical Data and Safety Monitoring Board, an independent panel set up by investigators that monitors clinical trials for any unexpected effects that might require a halt in the trial earlier than planned. Visco herself eventually took a position as a consumer representative on the steering committee that oversaw the entire Her-2/neu program.

John Curd views the interaction with the activists as a "positive growth experience" for the company: "We didn't want to do this. It costs money. It takes time. It takes effort. It's a diversion. It slows the progress of our clinical trials. But we began to understand something that we heard from one of the women [in ACT-UP] in one of the first meetings, that it is not all just an intellectual argument: 'Some of this is an emotional argument, and for those of us who are dealing with breast cancer or people who we know and love and have breast cancer, it's an emotional issue. We need to know that you are going to do something—not everything, but something.' "

When Genentech began phase III trials of the Her-2/neu antibody in 1995, it broke ground on a $300 million manufacturing plant that would produce the Her-2/neu drug. By coincidence, that plant is located in Vacaville, so close to Bob Erwin's house that he sees it every time he looks out his living room window. Also visible through that window is a new Kaiser Permanente clinic, where Marti Nelson had planned to practice. Erwin believes the antibody would have allowed his wife to live longer, even if it would not have cured her.

He says he is reminded of this every time he looks out his window. "I think that I've gone from being angry and frustrated to turning the experience into a constructive, positive sort of mission," he says. Perhaps, he continues, he will be able to look back "sometime in the future, five, ten, twenty years from now, and say, 'Well, we accomplished a lot.' " Then he starts to cry. "I'd really like to know that part of Marti's legacy is that other people are better off."

CHAPTER 9

Trials and Errors

Cancer activists had indisputably won a great victory. That a disorganized band of breast-cancer activists like the members of BCA and ACT-UP/Golden Gate, joined later by Fran Visco and the National Breast Cancer Coalition, could wrest a significant concession from a large and intransigent corporation like Genentech was an enormous step forward for their cause. But the activists were a minor problem for Genentech compared with the anguish and delay that marked the company's preparations for the phase III trials.

The final phase of drug testing presents one of the most difficult challenges in medicine. It is staggeringly expensive to mount; endless logistical complexities usually push the cost well over $100 million. Given the expense of the phase III trials and their importance as the principal criterion for FDA approval, they can make or break small biotechnology companies. Pharmaceutical giants like Merck or Glaxo Wellcome are less vulnerable because they already have hundreds of products on the market, so each individual drug represents a smaller piece of their profit pie.

In May 1994, when Genentech was organizing the final phase of testing, it had only three products on the market. As an independent corporation, a failed trial might have vaporized it, but Roche owned 60 percent of the company. Security brought its own complications. Roche had an option to buy the remainder of Genentech's stock and had set a timetable and terms for possibly purchasing the rest. By an accident of timing, the Her-2/neu trial could determine in large measure the value of the outstanding shares. Genentech's officers, compensated largely through stock-option packages, stood to gain millions of dollars if the trial succeeded, but could lose money and their positions of corporate power if it failed.

Clinical trials are never sure things. No matter how good the laboratory, animal, and preliminary clinical results look, no one ever knows whether a treatment really works without unacceptable side effects before it is tested extensively in humans. Her-2/neu brought special challenges because despite many attempts, no one had successfully employed an antibody against cancer, and while scientists had been talking about it for almost two decades, no one had successfully tested a treatment aimed at a basic genetic alteration of cancer.

The company needed to recruit hundreds of doctors, win the approval of their hospitals, and, finally, motivate the doctors to persuade hundreds of patients to participate. But just when the company most needed to maintain order, it once again became arbitrary and befuddled, committing many procedural mistakes that would substantially delay the odyssey of Her-2/neu.

A big problem was that Genentech, even though it had been in existence for seventeen years, lacked expertise with clinical trials. Scientists at the biotechnology company could look down their noses at "big pharma." But among the things gigantic drug companies do well is carry out trials that prove forcefully whether a drug is safe and effective. Genentech simply did not have the experience. The FDA was desperate to approve its first product, a genetically engineered version of human growth hormone. The growth hormone then available was extracted from animal brains and was causing a human version of mad cow disease. Academic scientists, not Genentech, led the trials of its heart-attack treatment t-PA. Not that Genentech maintained a hands-off policy. A congressional subcommittee investigation found that Genentech gave at least one and probably many key investigators thousands of dollars' worth of stock options. Although the company and the doctors said the gifts never compromised the results, many other doctors denounced the practice. The only successful clinical trial the company had run itself was the test of its drug for the lung disease cystic fibrosis.

In addition, Genentech had never really recovered from the fiascoes with interferon and related products in the 1980s and early '90s. Because the company had then determined to abandon cancer treatment, no oncologists remained on the staff when they were needed for Her-2/neu. Responsibility for organizing the Her-2/neu trial fell to John Curd, a rheumatologist, and Tom Twaddell, a slow-talking gastroenterologist who was appointed leader of the twenty-person Her-2/neu clinical team. Nevertheless, both men had valuable experience in drug development: Curd had led clinical trials of several drugs at the Scripps Clinic in La Jolla; Twaddell had led the team at Glaxo Wellcome that tested Zofran, the most effective antidote to chemotherapy-induced nausea. But Twadell and Curd were not in charge. The critical questions of trial design fell to Genentech's chief executive officer and four or five key vice presidents, many of whom remained skeptical of Her-2/neu. "We were working in a program where I think the probability of success was viewed as not high early on," Twaddell says. In addition to daunting organizational challenges, he and Curd had to contend with internal discouragement and disparagement.

Even before formal planning began, the two men initiated extensive contacts with about a dozen of oncology's "thought leaders," some of whom had been involved in the phase II trials. Among those consulted were Larry Norton at Sloan Kettering;

Karen Antman, formerly with Harvard's Dana-Farber Cancer Institute and now at Columbia-Presbyterian Medical Center in New York; and Daniel Hayes, then with Dana-Farber. Dennis Slamon remained an adviser to Genentech for its entire Her-2 effort. Support from these experts for the phase III trial was even more important than their support during the earlier stages of testing. Having Norton and the others in its corner would give Genentech a head start in recruiting other oncologists to take part in the study and would provide some assurance that the most influential voices in breast-cancer treatment would not attack Genentech later on in the process. Genentech paid them a standard consulting fee of several thousand dollars per day, and Twaddell and Curd kept them apprised of developments in the trial design, calling them often, visiting them, and gathering them for periodic "investigators' meetings."

Dealing with these gargantuan egos required tact. The participants were all substantial academic physicians, and their views were strongly held and often widely divergent. Even among this group, Larry Norton and a handful of others wielded significant influence. When Norton could not attend one meeting near the San Francisco International Airport, Twaddell passed around New York Mets caps as he related Norton's view to the participants. (Twaddell evidently believed in the talismanic powers of baseball caps. At the same meeting, he distributed Astros caps as he described the views of another influential player, Gabriel Hortobagyi of M. D. Anderson Cancer Center in Houston.)

The coddling did not guarantee unanimity. At one investigators' meeting, Craig Henderson of UCSF, often contrarian and combative, offered his own plan for an extremely complicated trial. Curd looked around the room and thought that everyone agreed with Henderson. He soon realized that the others were staring off into space or at their shoes and had stopped listening. Disagreements notwithstanding, a fairly consistent view emerged that the tests should take place in women newly diagnosed with breast-cancer metastases, a group whose disease is relatively treatable compared with cancers in even later stages. Companies traditionally test new cancer drugs in patients with much more advanced diseases and fewer options for treatments. If those tests have optimistic results, then doctors try it on patients at earlier and earlier stages. No company had ever tested a breast-cancer drug in the newly diagnosed population because most doctors did not want to use an unproved therapy on patients in the early, more treatable stages of the disease. But because the antibody appeared to be nontoxic, testing it at an earlier stage appeared justified. Moreover, the outside experts and many Genentech officials felt that if the antibody proved useful at all, it would be as a means of holding the cancer in check while chemotherapy attacked it. They felt that women with early-stage disease could best demonstrate those effects.

But the phase II trials had yielded a big surprise. They were meant to test for possible effectiveness, but no one expected the antibody by itself to shrink tumors, let alone bring about spectacular cancer remissions, like Mary Bonesco's. Still, despite the good results, the investigators agreed that the use of an antibody alone remained too new a concept to test on women in relatively early stages of the disease. Existing chemotherapy regimens could successfully treat (if not ultimately cure) newly metastatic breast cancer. The doctors thought it would be unethical to deny chemotherapy treatment to patients in the trial. So the question became, Which chemotherapy to use in combination with the antibody? Half the phase II trials studied the antibody with cisplatin, the combination that had cured Barbara Bradfield.

But the consultants opposed any further tests with the controversial combination that Slamon had championed. As Curd recalls it, "The very same people who told us that it would be a good combination to take into phase III turned around and said, 'I can't give my patients cisplatin because it's not active in breast cancer.' " The "thought leaders" had voiced few objections to an early trial of the antibody with cisplatin. It involved only a few advanced patients. But now, when they considered enrolling large numbers of patients for the pivotal trial, different considerations emerged. Everyone knew that cisplatin by itself could not treat breast cancer. The "thought leaders" would not risk putting large numbers of patients with less-advanced disease on a combination of agents where one, the antibody, was highly experimental and the other, cisplatin, was useless by itself. Without patients, Genentech would never get the answer it needed about the Her-2/neu antibody.

Dennis Slamon was livid. Both he and Mike Shepard had gotten lab results demonstrating the power of the cisplatin-antibody combination, but now Genentech was walking away from positive clinical results that included Barbara Bradfield's complete response. No one supported Slamon's passionate belief that the phase III trials should test the antibody with cisplatin. In his zeal to prove that his treatment worked, Slamon wanted to try what he thought best immediately. But his fellow physicians were willing to risk only a much more gradual change in practice. He was "the Lone Ranger in this issue," says Twaddell. Slamon and his small gang of Genentech loyalists in the Research Department had held such sway with the company three years before, but now they were viewed as malcontents.

A strategy emerged to treat every patient in the group with CA, Cytoxan and Adriamycin, the major chemotherapy combination for metastatic breast cancer, and give half of them Her-2/neu. Larry Norton, however, offered another suggestion. He was involved in ongoing tests of Taxol for breast cancer, and although all the results were not in, he believed it worked well. Moreover, his junior associate, José Baselga, had carried out lab tests showing that the Taxol-antibody combination worked far better than the CA-antibody combination.

Curd and Twaddell formally suggested to management that it carry out a double trial to test CA with and without antibody and Taxol with and without antibody. When management refused to support two separate trials, the two men suggested a large, simple trial. Participating oncologists would treat their patients with whatever conventional treatment they chose, and in addition they would give half their patients antibody. This approach had proved successful for winning approval of cardiac and AIDS medications, but it left the Genentech staff who dealt with the FDA very nervous. They would need to test too many patients and perform statistical calculations that were overwhelmingly complex.

Management scaled back the trial to a comparison of CA and antibody with CA and placebo. Curd and Twaddell opposed the decision and were frustrated by how little influence they had on it. "It was very difficult for me to really know what truly went on behind the scenes," says Twaddell. Curd says that Twaddell and his team "knew damn good and well it was going to be hard [to carry out the trial], and they [told] the company it's really going to be hard. The company was not listening."

Art Levinson, now Genentech's chief executive officer, paints a different picture. While he readily concedes that the company's early management style—before he took over—could be chaotic, he says that the planning of phase III trials, in which he played a key role as senior vice president for research, proceeded in an orderly fashion. Three years later, when there was ample evidence that the drug had overcome the trial-design difficulties and would be successful, Levinson said, "It might be easy for people now in retrospect to say, 'Oh, I could tell you this trial was going to be difficult.' I was part of every one of those [Product Development Committee] meetings that talked about phase III trial design, and I cannot remember anybody saying, 'This is a flawed study' or 'We won't be able to enroll it.' If anybody had that opinion, it was never expressed around the table. It would have been foolish of us to spend all the money we spent on a trial that wasn't going to enroll. What would be the rationale of doing something like that?"

As the trials got under way, many people started asking precisely that question. Part of the answer seemed to be Genentech's legacy of confused management and its lack of experience with clinical trials. Larry Norton, for one, thought the trial design was terribly flawed. In fact, he felt snubbed because Genentech had rejected his Taxol suggestion, and he did not hesitate to express his resentment to anyone interested.

As drug trials proceed, each phase incorporates knowledge gained from the one before. But Genentech management was proposing a radically different and risky approach. "We did not have a phase II program that said our drug would work in phase III," says Curd. He suggested a new phase II study of the antibody-CA combination in fifty patients, but his proposal met with rejection. Most large drug companies would have ordered a feasibility study, a second phase II study with the new combination, before embarking on the massive expense and risk of phase III. The planners were even confused about what dose of antibody they should administer. Much of the dose information they gained from the earlier trials came from correlating the antibody dose with cisplatin. Now they were combining the antibody with other chemotherapy agents, and it might turn out they were using less than the optimum dose. But Genentech management was in a hurry to start the trial. The Roche buyout timetable may have played a role, though Levinson denied that it had anything to do with the decision. "This drug alone is not going to be the determinant of what our stock price is going to be," he said. Curiously, management spent another six months arguing about the specifics of the trial—about the amount of time that it would have taken to carry out a second phase II study.

Finally, in January 1995, Twaddell finished writing the detailed protocols that would be submitted to the FDA for the approval required to test the Her-2/neu antibody in phase III trials. In the pivotal trial, called 648 (Genentech, like most drug companies, assigns sequential numbers to its clinical trials), 450 women with newly diagnosed metastatic breast cancer were to be randomly divided into two groups. Half would get CA plus the Her-2/neu antibody and the others, CA plus infusions of saline solution, a dummy medication. Neither the doctor nor the patient would know who was getting the antibody and who was not. This design—known as double blind placebo controlled—is the gold standard of clinical trials. Wishful thinking cannot influence the results. Thus, data from such a trial offer the most definitive scientific evidence. The FDA had pushed for the placebo because it had little experience with antibodies as cancer treatments and wanted data that would be the easiest to interpret. The double-blind-placebo-controlled study offered the best chance of proving conclusively that the antibody worked. But cancer-drug trials had never employed a placebo before. How could they? Cancer drugs left people nauseated and bald. Everyone would know who was getting the drug.

To try to answer some of the questions that the panel of experts had debated, Genentech added two smaller trials of two hundred women each. Trial 649 administered antibody alone to women whose metastatic disease had failed to respond to one or two rounds of chemotherapy. Trial 650 offered antibody alone to women who had newly metastatic disease but did not want any chemotherapy. By mid-1995, all the pieces were finally in place to test the new breast-cancer treatment, but the effort immediately faltered. "I would tell you in retrospect," John Curd says, "the team was sent on a mission to Antarctica without a coat."

Failure to Accrue

As the trials got under way, Genentech's Marketing Department moved to find a name for the new treatment. Companies regard naming as an extraordinarily serious matter. The name attracts physician and patient recognition that can make a huge difference in sales. Drugs and biological treatments carry two names—the generic and the trade name. For drugs, the generic name is often simply that of the chemical that makes up the drug. But for biological products like a laboratory-created antibody, a government agency assigns a name that includes a required prefix and suffix with some seemingly random vowels and consonants in between. For the Her-2/neu antibody, that name was Trastuzumab, hardly destined to flow off many tongues. To come up with the trade name that everyone would eventually use, the marketing people first asked for suggestions from the Her-2 clinical team. The name should reflect some of the science, and from the outset everyone assumed it would begin with *Her* because of the gene's name and the obvious connection to a woman's disease. Members of the clinical team decided to emphasize the antibody's inhibition of cancerous growth and suggested Herhibon.

The marketing people, not quite satisfied, turned to Interbrand of New York, whose core business is naming drugs. Interbrand came back with Tarcepton—intercepting the target—and the Genentech Marketing Department decided on combining the two suggestions: Herceptin. Genentech next asked its "thought leaders" for their opinion and paid Interbrand to set up focus groups of oncologists and physicians with other specialties to test their responses to Herceptin as well as other candidates. Most important, both Interbrand and Genentech's Legal Department undertook an extensive search to find out whether the name meant something offensive in any language and whether anyone had ever tried to copyright any part of it.

To establish the massive infrastructure needed to conduct the large, complicated trial of Herceptin and recruit most of the doctors needed to carry it out, Genentech turned to Corning Besselaar, a drug-contract research organization. A few large drug companies still maintain clinical departments with a large enough staff to organize phase III trials, but to avoid the hassle of hiring hundreds of temporary employees, small companies like Genentech hire contractors like Corning Besselaar. In many cases, the arrangement works well, but it puts another layer of bureaucracy between the drug company and the physicians who play the most crucial role.

Over the first half of 1995, Corning Besselaar set up ninety-nine sites in the United States, seven in Canada, thirty-three in Europe, ten in Australia, and one in New Zealand to carry out the Her-2/ neu tests. The physicians carrying out phase III cancer-drug trials often work a notch below the superstars at large academic medical centers. More prominent physicians prefer to attach their names to the more prestigious phase I and phase II trials, which provide greater opportunity for publishing important research papers even though they do not prove definitively whether a drug works. Doctors who conduct phase III trials tend to practice in less well known institutions or at hospitals with no academic affiliation. A few work in private practice.

For doctors, phase III trials have their attractions even if they don't promise professional recognition. Genentech and other drug companies reimburse the doctors for patient visits for the tests and for all time spent doing the required record keeping. But the money alone seldom interests the doctors. For the most part, they want to offer their patients something beyond the standard regimens and to gain a reputation for doing so. For Her-2/neu, more than 150 doctors stood ready to enroll the required 450 patients in the key trial, number 648, the double-blind-placebo-controlled study. But as Twaddell and his team waited for patients to enroll, they got almost none.

The 649 trial filled its slots more rapidly. This was hardly surprising since it represented more of a last hope for women whose cancer had failed to respond to chemotherapy. But at the beginning, even enrolling in that trial could be difficult.

Ginger Empey, a nurse from Bakersfield, California, learned she had breast cancer in February 1995 and that it already had metastasized to her liver and spine. She tried CAF and Taxol, but they did nothing. With a great deal of difficulty, as she recalls, she persuaded her hometown oncologist to refer her to UCLA for high-dose chemotherapy with bone-marrow rescue. But the UCLA doctors determined that her tumor remained so resistant to chemotherapy that she was ineligible for the high-dose regime. In June a young colleague of John Glaspy on the transplant team at UCLA told her: "I suggest you take a trip, do whatever you want, do whatever you can. Get your affairs in order."

Empey, who is so energetic and youthful in appearance that people often assume her grandchildren are her children, was not about to accept the death sentence. She told the young doctor, "I cannot believe that at this fabulous institution that there is not something else, that there is not some other treatment, there is not some clinical trial—something here for me." Finally the doctor told her, "Oh, well, there is a trial that's opening up pretty soon, but it's pretty hard to qualify, and I doubt you will." He said he would have someone call her. She wrote down the name of the drug. It was Her-2/neu.

Empey returned to the Rhonda Fleming Mann Resource Center for Women with Breast Cancer at UCLA. She had been there before in search of research and a support group. Now she asked specifically about Her-2/neu. They told her Slamon had given a talk there and they gave her a tape of it that she played on her long car ride home. "This is for me. I'm doing it," she decided.

Empey was not someone who waited meekly for a telephone call. She got the number of the clinical coordinator at UCLA and arranged to have her tumor block shipped there. She was highly positive for Her-2/neu. "I was just thrilled," she says. "I was a hot one. I wanted treatment." But things did not move as quickly as she wanted. At every hospital, a committee called the Institutional Review Board must approve all experiments on humans, including all clinical trials. But the committee at UCLA was having trouble granting the formal permission. It was summer and the committee's members, doctors and nurses, were on vacation. Empey refused to sit still.

"I drove them crazy. I called them twice a week, every week. What did the human subjects committee come up with? Do you have the consent? Is the nurse still on vacation? Is her house remodeled? I mean, I just, I was *awful*." And this was UCLA—Dennis Slamon's hospital—with a resource center where one could hear a tape of Slamon explaining the treatment! Empey finally got her approval and became the first patient in phase III. She got her first infusion, the first treatment in the phase III trial, on August 31, 1995. Gradually, her tumors shrank. By Christmas 1995 she recalls, "I felt like I had gotten my life back again."

Other women around the world began to make their way to the 649 trial fairly quickly. But the 648 trial was a different matter. In

June 1995, one woman signed up. In July, a second patient enrolled. By the end of October 1995, a total of fourteen women around the world had signed up. Why were patients just trickling in? It was not just that the process of enrollment was difficult. Plenty of oncologists, especially leading academics, were disturbed that the phase III study did not follow from phase II. As Curd puts it, "They're looking at this and saying Genentech's reaching."

Since this was the first trial ever to test a drug in women with newly metastatic disease, the planners had failed to appreciate another dimension. Most of the women received their care not in academic medical centers but from their local oncologists. To enroll a patient in a trial, doctors would have to relinquish that patient to the closest participating hospital, often many miles away, and forfeit the income that she would bring. Curd understands the doctors' dilemma. Genentech was asking them "to turn their patients over to someone and in effect say, 'I don't know exactly who he is. He's got an experimental regimen. He's going to give you the same stuff I'm gonna give you, plus something else.' So right away you can't really take care of your patient. It's inconvenient for your patient. And you lose revenue."

These were not the hopeless cases a doctor might send to a big medical center when he had nothing left to offer. These were cases where the doctor could offer proven treatments. Not cures, to be sure, but drugs that could add months or even years to a woman's life. Indeed, because breast cancer strikes so often and because oncologists could offer their patients known treatments, metastatic breast cancer had become the bread and butter for most oncologists. Furthermore, doctors willing to consider experimental treatment for a patient had more than Her-2/neu to consider. Bone-marrow transplants were gaining favor, and if a community oncologist was inclined to send the woman to a hospital for treatment for newly metastatic disease, it would likely be for high-dose chemotherapy with bone-marrow rescue.

Another reason for doctors' reluctance to enroll patients in the trial was Her-2/neu's narrow effectiveness. Because only 25 to 30 percent of breast-cancer cases test positive for Her-2/neu, doctors suggesting the treatment stood a good chance of setting their patients up for disappointment. Some doctors reported referring eight or nine cases in a row whose Her-2/neu results came back negative. Doctors concluded that it simply did not add up to a worthwhile effort.

The situation suggested the terrifying possibility that the trial would fail. Larry Norton says that for a clinical trial to succeed, "there has to be a ground swell of interest in it. And that has to build up an enormous accrual right away that then carries it through to completion, to the end of the trial. If you have a trial that you design that sort of inches along, a certain pessimism develops about the trial itself that is self-perpetuating. And nobody wants to go on a trial that isn't going anywhere. No doctor wants to include a patient in a trial that isn't going anywhere." Almost from the moment of inception, it was clear the trial was going nowhere and that no matter how many lives the treatment might save, it might never reach the women who needed it.

Genentech soon realized that the biggest obstacle to enrollment was the placebo. The women would get CA in any case, but doctors did not want their patients to face the possibility that they might not get the experimental drug that might save their lives. Although few of the "thought leaders" raised objections to the placebo when the study was planned, they seemed to have little sympathy for Genentech's problems when they arose. "The very same people who had advised us on this told us, well, they wouldn't enroll the patients in it because oncologists don't want to have patients on placebo," says Curd. "One of the good things about being a 'thought leader' is you can change your mind." Most cancer doctors simply refused to submit their patients to the possibility that they would face what Kathy Crooks endured.

Kathy Crooks is a supremely self-confident and tough woman. She lives with her husband, Larry Hartman, and their son, Devin, in suburban Glen Ellyn, Illinois. A past president of the local chapter of the National Organization for Women, Crooks runs her own business distributing janitorial supplies for factories, simultaneously managing, as she puts it, "home, child, and business." She remembers when Devin, who is now twelve, was an infant she would be taking orders on the phone and the customers would hear the sound of her nursing her son. "Kathy, what *is* that noise?" she remembers the men asking. "And I would tell them, 'That's Devin having lunch.' And there would be a long silence on the other end, but they placed the order anyway. So it was really a riot."

When she needed medical care Crooks had no hesitation about taking charge. She was diagnosed with inflammatory breast cancer in 1994 at age forty-three. Inflammatory breast cancer is a rare form of the disease that causes the skin to turn red or orange and the breast to swell rapidly. It spreads with unusual speed. Her-2/neu positive tumors often take this form. The treatment usually involves chemotherapy first, followed by surgery, followed by more chemotherapy and radiation.

Crooks sought treatment at Rush-Presbyterian-St. Luke's Medical Center in Chicago. Melody Cobleigh, a mild-mannered, extraordinarily warm breast-cancer specialist, took her case and immediately put her on the maximum number of chemotherapy drugs, a mixture the nurses called the garbage-pizza treatment. She underwent a lumpectomy, which failed to get all of the tumor, followed in February 1995 by a modified radical mastectomy. The surgeon had discovered twelve cancerous lymph nodes. More chemotherapy and radiation followed.

A thorough physical examination in October 1995 showed Crooks to be cancer free, and she relaxed a bit. But only four months later a nagging cough sent her to the doctor. Cobleigh was off attending a medical conference, so Crooks saw an internist in her neighborhood who ordered a chest X ray. Crooks remembers the doctor's reaction when she saw the film. "She freaked out on me. She literally freaked out on me. She said, 'Your lungs look like Christmas trees.'" At first, Crooks could not believe the cancer had returned so rapidly.

"This was the Andromeda strain," Cobleigh recalls.

As it turned out Cobleigh was not just one of the investigators for Her-2 but one its most enthusiastic backers. "I hate chemotherapy," she says. She thought Herceptin represented Kathy Crook's best chance. Crooks signed up for the 648 trial, which treated women with either the Her-2/neu antibody or placebo, plus chemotherapy. Fourteen other women were in the study at that time in the same hospital. Crooks got her chemotherapy infusion every third Friday. Each Tuesday, she went in to receive the Her-2/neu antibody or placebo—she did not know which, and neither did the doctors or nurses. Early on, Crooks suspected that she was getting the placebo because the antibody, though nontoxic by the standards of chemo-therapy, caused flulike symptoms in some women or soreness at the site of their cancer during the first dose. The infusion room gossip had wrongly assumed that all women on the antibody developed symptoms. In fact, the data would show that 40 percent did. "I knew it wasn't Her-2 because I knew I would feel something. I knew it would be an improvement," Crooks said.

After several weeks—by early May—it was obvious to the doc-tors and nurses that there was no improvement in Crooks's condi-tion, and they were getting nervous. "They came over and looked at me, and I said, 'You know, I really should tell you I'm not breath-ing too well anymore,'" she recalls. Says Cobleigh, "She was dying in front of our eyes."

Under the 648 protocol, if a woman's cancer did not improve or if it got worse over an eight-week period, the doctor could seek Genentech's permission to make certain the patient was getting antibody and not placebo. But switching a patient from placebo to antibody often required days or weeks of paperwork. In fact, that delay brought yet another criticism of the trial. Cobleigh did not think Crooks had the time, so she phoned Genentech. No one there could quickly find the information that would have told her whether Crooks was getting the placebo. She had a final resort: the labels on the placebo and on the antibody had a tiny square covered with scratch-off material like that covering the numbers on a lottery ticket. Only in extreme emergencies, like suspected poisoning, were doctors supposed to scratch off the square to reveal the contents of the infusion bag. But Cobleigh scratched it off and learned that Crooks was getting placebo. She immediately phoned Genentech and asked how quickly she could get antibody for Crooks. It arrived the next morning.

Kathy Crooks got her first infusion, known as the loading dose, and in about one hour she started to shake all over. She describes the symptom as DTs. When she got home that evening, she could barely drag herself to bed. She tried to eat a slice of bread, but it came right back up. By 8:00 P.M., she started to feel a little better, and by 10:00 P.M. she was fine. In the morning, she called the oncology nurse who worked with Cobleigh and described what happened. The nurse responded, "Wonderful! That's great! We have a theory: the worse you feel, the better you're doing on the drug."

By the second or third dose, she thought she felt an improvement. By the fourth dose, she was definitely breathing more easily. "Every week, you just start getting better and better and better," she says. Her first set of scans, twelve weeks into the Her-2/neu infusions, showed that her tumors were shrinking. The medical staff was stunned by the progress. "It was phenomenal. They were absolutely hanging off the rafters, they were so happy," says Crooks. "It was one of the most astounding recoveries I have ever seen," says Cobleigh.

All along, her family and friends had been against her participating in the randomized study. Their fear had been that she'd go through all the discomfort of infusions and end up getting saline instead of the drug. "It was very stressful," recalls Crooks, "because you have the survivors and the nonsurvivors, and you're sitting side by side" in the infusion room. But Crooks figured going in that it was a no-lose situation. "Once I'm in this protocol," she argued, "they can't deny me if I need it. I made sure that as long as I paid my dues, I was going to get it. So I paid my dues for six weeks." Because her doctor was willing to act quickly, she did end up getting Her-2/neu but just in the nick of time. It was a case that could easily have gone badly, and that's what scared off oncologists.

As Tom Twaddell worked furiously to rally his staff and network of doctors, he realized with increasing despair that major changes would be needed if the trial were to stand any chance of success. One of his biggest concerns was his impression that Corning Besselaar did not take the project seriously enough to assign it its best staff. "I think that they had some good people on the project, but it didn't start well," Twaddell recalls. Curiously, the trial did accrue patients in places like Australia, presumably because the contractor's representative there evidenced some enthusiasm. But in the United States and especially in Europe, the effort lagged. The Her-2 phase III trials should have been attracting large numbers of volunteers, but so few appeared that the trial was in danger of closing down. One problem was that while Corning Besselaar had run several clinical trials, the company had little experience with cancer drugs and few contacts in the world of oncology. Moreover, Genentech had promised to give Corning Besselaar a set amount of business, which left Twaddell out of the loop in setting up the arrangement and unable to mend what he saw as key problems at the outset. "I didn't have control over the arrangement with the contract research organization," he says, "which is clearly not a circumstance that I would work under again."

CHAPTER 11

Strawberries and Champagne

For months, Genentech's board of directors had been dissatisfied with the company's chief executive, Kirk Raab. Raab had never been a fan of the Her-2/neu effort, but that was hardly the problem. One complaint centered on a $2 million loan guarantee for a new home that Raab had allegedly demanded from Roche during his secret talks to renegotiate the terms for the takeover of the outstanding Genentech stock. He said he simply needed the cash to buy the house, but Roche officers reportedly found the demand offensive, especially since stockholders' lawsuits charged that Raab had given Roche a sweet deal. But the larger problem was Raab's management style, his emphasis on intensive and sometimes questionable marketing efforts. On his watch, Genentech's efforts to sell growth hormone and t-PA led to several federal investigations. On July 10, 1995, the board ousted him and gave his job to Art Levinson, who promised to restore integrity to the company's business practices.

The scientific staff at Genentech—including the Her-2/neu team—was thrilled to have one of their own at the helm. Levinson had trained as a cancer researcher, first as a graduate student at Princeton, then as a postdoctoral fellow in the laboratory of

Michael Bishop, who had found the first oncogene. Levinson's own research focused on oncogenes. He even played a role in helping Axel Ullrich clone the Her-2/neu gene, earning coauthor's position on the paper in *Nature* detailing the achievement. As he moved up in management, Levinson rescued the Her-2/neu project from extinction on several occasions.

In November 1995, Genentech management decided to implement the first major change in the phase III effort. To draw more participants to 648, it took Larry Norton's suggestion and added Taxol to the protocol as an alternative to Adriamycin, opening up the protocol to women whose cancers had already failed to respond to Adriamycin. Until that point, the trial participants were getting CA—Cytoxan and Adriamycin—along with either antibody or placebo.

More than one hundred women ultimately volunteered for the Taxol arm of the 648 trial, and the results would prove critical. But it was the last change during Twaddell's tenure. He had led a failing effort, and his staff was thoroughly demoralized. Genentech management had already placed much of the blame for the troubled trial on him. It was one of the worst periods of his professional life. "But it's the hand we get dealt," he says. Early in 1996, Genentech took him off the clinical trial. It was an invitation for him to look for work elsewhere.

John Curd did not lose his position, but Genentech brought in someone with experience in breast-cancer-therapy research to oversee him. Susan Hellmann, a thirty-eight-year-old oncologist, took over supervision of the trial. Hellmann had worked at Bristol-Myers Squibb, where she had been a part of the team that initially tested Taxol in ovarian cancer and then in breast cancer. For the first time since interferon, Genentech seemed to be taking cancer treatment seriously.

The impetus for a total overhaul of the Her-2/neu trials occurred not in Genentech headquarters on the shores of San Francisco Bay but in a dark, paneled room of the Harvard Club in Manhattan. Larry Norton, despite whatever reservations he might have had at one time about Her-2/neu, remained angry about what he saw as the poor design of the clinical trial. Norton barely knew David Botstein, who had served as Genentech vice president for clinical research and remained as a company consultant. Both men served as directors of a biotech company called Amplicon, which was holding a board meeting at the Harvard Club in January 1996. Norton, who did not think the Taxol option was enough to fix the trial, approached Botstein with an earful. "The Her-2/neu trial is all fucked up," Norton said. "It's like an octopus so complicated no one can figure it out, and it will never accrue." Botstein quickly arranged for Norton to speak with with Susan Hellmann. Hellmann, who had become vice president for clinical affairs, assuming responsibility for the entire Her-2 effort, remembers that in the first few conversations Norton did not speak to her. He was so angry about the manner in which the trials had been conducted that he only screamed. "I thought I was beginning to make great progress with Larry," she remembers, "when he started to talk to me in a normal tone of voice." She quickly made sure that top management heard Norton's views.

Hank Fuchs, irreverent and often rumpled, took Twaddell's job as head of the Her-2/neu project in February 1996. Thirty-nine years old at the time, the fast-talking physician was already a star at Genentech and in the early 1990s had run clinical trials for Pulmozyme, a treatment for cystic fibrosis. Working with patient-advocacy groups and with Corning Besselaar, Fuchs had sailed the trial flawlessly to FDA approval.

In fact, FDA Commissioner David Kessler had unusually high praise for the effort. "It was a large trial, it had clinical endpoints of statistical power, and it was able to demonstrate unequivocally that the drug worked. Sometimes we see twenty-five trials on a drug, and in the end we have more questions than answers," Kessler told

The New York Times. When Fuchs took over the Her-2/neu project, he did not encounter the same problems with the contractor that had hampered Twaddell's efforts. Fuchs enjoyed a good relationship with Corning Besselaar. He worked with the company both on the cystic fibrosis trial and on a trial that tested Pulmozyme as a treatment for the much more common condition called chronic obstructive lung disease. The drug was not effective in this case, but most agreed that Fuchs had run the trial well.

Fuchs had never intended to work for a drug company. The son of a physician, he grew up in Bethesda, Maryland, in the shadow of the National Institutes of Health. While he was a sophomore at Harvard, his twenty-nine-year-old brother, Dan, was diagnosed with a malignant brain tumor. Three years later Hank remembers standing outside his dying brother's hospital room at George Washington University Hospital and thinking, "I hope that everybody here is spending all their time working on this." He attended Washington University Medical School and took a postdoctoral fellowship at UCSF in 1985. He moved to Genentech two years later for what he thought would be a brief stay to carry out basic research supported by the California Lung Association. There he happened to share a lab bench with one of the scientists working on the Her-2/neu project. He became fascinated with the possibilities and challenges of drug research.

In early 1996, few efforts in drug development could have presented more of a challenge than the moribund Her-2/neu effort. Fuchs had to set the trial on the right course. "How do you unwind time?" Fuchs asked. His first act was to visit many of the doctors throughout the United States and Europe who had volunteered to conduct the tests, asking their opinion on redesigning the trial. Courting the oncologists, he felt, was the key to kick-starting the trials, and he put his energy into "reengaging their hearts and minds."

To Fuchs's way of thinking, if the doctors weren't enthusiastic, then the patients would never come on board. "The [patient's] decision to participate in clinical trials is made right in the first four seconds, according to what the doctor says," he explained. "If the doctor says, 'Why the hell are you going to do this?' then it's an overwhelming barrier to overcome. If the doctor says, 'I really think you need to think about a clinical trial,' then it's practically a slam dunk."

A month into his new job, Fuchs redesigned the phase III protocols. Most significantly, he dropped the placebo from the key 648 trial. The participants would still be randomized, but doctors and patients would know who was getting the antibody and who was not. He also streamlined the enrollment process. Twaddell and his team had argued for many of these same changes, but management had refused to permit them. The situation had simply not been dire enough for such moves. As Curd puts it, "If the team had tried to do what Hank did a year sooner, they would have gotten the classical sort of management techniques: bullet points, no bonus, those kinds of things. You would have been non–team players. So it was really different. We got to where Hank was because we were desperate."

To implement the new procedures, Fuchs needed at least the tacit approval of the FDA, referred to in somber tones as "The Agency" by people who work in drug companies. The FDA, after all, had been insistent on the placebo. To head off the criticism that doing away with it would prejudice the way doctors measured the data, Fuchs set up an independent panel of radiologists to monitor patient MRIs and other scans. The panelists would not know who was getting the antibody; they would not even know a patient's age or her medical history. They would only measure and compare the size of tumors on different dates.

Genentech had already had a memorably negative experience with the FDA. In May 1987, an FDA advisory panel had denied the company's application to market what became its biggest product: Activase, or t-PA, a clot dissolver to treat heart attacks. Many peo-

ple thought that Genentech had arrogantly and stupidly ignored
FDA requests for information. After an extensive Genentech-
sponsored lobbying campaign, FDA commissioner Frank Young
took the unusual step of overruling his advisory panel and approved t-PA in November of that year. But the delay cost Genentech dearly. "Genentech, particularly through its experience with
t-PA, learned that it's very important to listen frequently and carefully to what the FDA says," says Curd.

Fuchs could not have picked a better time to seek the FDA's ab-
solution. Michael Friedman, a huge teddy bear of a man with a
full beard and a soft-spoken Southern accent, had recently joined
the agency as deputy commissioner. In a few months, he would
become acting commissioner. An oncologist who had been on the
faculty of UCSF, he had spent eight years as director of the
treatment-evaluation program at the National Cancer Institute,
and he cared deeply about the effort to improve cancer treatments. On March 29, 1996, he achieved a goal for which he had
lobbied since his arrival at FDA: he stood in the East Room of the
White House as President Bill Clinton announced that the FDA
would streamline its approval for cancer drugs. "The waiting is
over," declared the president, whose mother had recently died of
breast cancer. "We cannot guarantee miracles, but at least now
new hope is on the way."

The announcement was the culmination of an FDA effort that
had quietly been under way since about 1990. For many years, the
FDA, working with the pharmaceutical giants, had approved drugs
through an unwieldy and complicated bureaucratic process. It was
like two hippopotamuses dancing a slow waltz. The process per-
fectly suited the conservative companies, whose business depends
not on speed but on a steady, reliable stream of new products. But
biotechnology companies, whose very existence often requires the
approval of a single drug, lobbied for rapid approval, which almost
always follows successful completion of phase III trials. Coinci-

dentally, AIDS activists were working toward the same goal, staging noisy and confrontational demonstrations to light a fire under the FDA bureaucracy.

Under the new rules, companies need no longer prove that a cancer drug improves survival or even quality of life. They simply must show that it shrinks tumors, even if only temporarily. "We've got to have mechanisms in place to speed up the development to the shortest possible time between when you first think of using [a new drug], first put it into the first patient, and when you have enough information to say that it's ready for general use," Friedman said soon after Clinton's announcement.

Clinton's move formalized a change in practice initiated several years earlier by FDA commissioner David Kessler, who fought to speed up the drug-approval process. The first example of accelerated approval for a cancer drug came in December 1992, when the FDA gave Bristol-Myers the nod to market Taxol. Studies showed that the drug reduced tumors in about 30 percent of women with highly advanced ovarian cancer, but the effect lasted an average of only six months before the life-threatening cancer began to grow again—hardly a dramatic cure. But after the approval, successive studies showed that if administered early in the course of ovarian cancer (as well as breast cancer), Taxol could yield far more dramatic results.

Revamping the FDA's bureaucracy was no easy matter. Most of the staff of seven hundred who review new applications for new drugs and the four hundred who review biologics (the heading under which the antibody falls) are meticulous, dedicated civil servants who often work for a fraction of what they could make in the private sector. They perceive themselves as defenders of the public health even as they feel besieged by a public and politicians who fail to appreciate their effort. "It's very hard to turn this battleship in the river" is how Drug Division head Robert Temple puts it.

At first, the FDA reacted coolly to Genentech's bid to drop the placebo and initiate other changes in the trial. According to Curd, the FDA said, "By dropping the placebo, you're taking risks with your trial. And we said, 'Yes, we understand.' " Curd said the FDA officials warned that if the lack of placebo appeared to influence the results, Genentech would have to repeat the study, and "to a company like Genentech that's like driving a stake through the heart." Given the trial's stagnant performance up to then, however, Genentech had to make some sort of radical change, and it was willing to take the risk. With the placebo in place, the trial would clearly fail.

In the spring of 1996, Genentech mailed the new protocols, the new rules for the trials, to the more than 150 sites. But enrollment continued to lag. From June 1995 until the end of the year, only twenty-one women had signed on for the 648 trial. In the first five months of 1996, about a dozen women a month volunteered, an increase. But even at that rate, it would have taken until 1999 to accrue the needed 450 patients, and the results would not have been known until 2000. "We're sucking wind here," Fuchs said on June 6 at a strategic planning session at the Hotel Plaza Athenee in Manhattan. Attending the meeting was Bruce Teplitzky, the easygoing head of Corning Besselaar's Her-2/neu operation. Fuchs, who had already had good experiences dealing with the contractor, had little trouble working with Teplitzky to implement the changes.

The two men brought together a staff totaling a dozen women, the foot soldiers in the U.S. and European clinical-trial effort, and the team hammered out a detailed plan to whip up more interest among the doctors and attract more women to volunteer. It was a multipronged effort. Representatives were to fan out across the country to tell investigators about the changes in the trial and to offer whatever help they could in attracting patients. A few weeks later, Fuchs recruited Slamon for a six-city tour. In each location,

Genentech paid the expenses for the regional investigators to attend a daylong symposium, where they heard Fuchs and others describe changes in the trial. Slamon once again set out the scientific rationale. In addition, Genentech's Public Relations Department sent informational materials and offered assistance to any hospital that wished to hold a press conference announcing that the trial was open. The company even prepared all-purpose press releases so hospital public-relations staffs would only have to fill in a few blanks, and it sent out videotapes so local TV stations would have pictures to go with the story.

Fuchs also tried to attract more community oncologists to the trial, enlisting the aid of academic oncologists like Debu Tripathey, who were already enthusiastically involved. Genentech arranged for the academics to host dinner meetings with colleagues in their communities. Similarly, the company tried to plug into existing networks connecting academic oncologists to doctors in private practice. Using mostly Revlon money, Slamon had already set up a program in southern California to send nurses into the field to help local oncologists carry out Her-2/neu and other clinical trials. The nurses, who met regularly at UCLA to learn the latest developments in all the trial procedures, brought the fresh information back to the doctors who were enrolling patients. Genentech tried to duplicate Slamon's system by hiring nurses to help oncologists around the country to participate in the clinical trial. This part of the effort, while ambitious, was hardly cheap. The salary and benefits for each nurse came to approximately fifty thousand dollars and yielded few extra patients.

What eventually did pay off, however, was the cooperation of the National Breast Cancer Coalition. Genentech forged the relationship first as a defensive response to the pressure from the activists in San Francisco. Over time, the relationship grew stronger. Genentech invited Visco to sit in as a consumer representative on its steering committee, the panel of outside experts that advised the company on its trial. Now it sought her help in urging local chapters to publicize the trials.

Again Genentech was taking a big risk. The company armed Visco's network with glossy brochures and videotapes describing the trials, a move that theoretically could have constituted illegal drug advertising. It was a charge that had stymied Genentech many times in the past. To market human growth hormone, the company had organized a campaign to measure millions of schoolchildren in the hope that parents or teachers would seek the hormone for short kids. The activities led to yet more federal investigations, and a Genentech vice president was indicted though eventually acquitted on charges of bribing doctors to prescribe growth hormone.

To avoid similar problems with Her-2/neu, Genentech turned to the lobbying firm of Bass and Howes, which had run interference for the company with the National Breast Cancer Coalition. In June 1966, Joanne Howes greased the wheels for a meeting at the FDA at which Fuchs and others detailed their plans to use the activist groups to make breast-cancer patients and their physicians aware of the trial. The FDA had no trouble with the proposal. Fuchs remembers the response as "How can we help you?"

Genentech mailed out two thousand brochures describing the Her-2/neu trial to all the groups and individual activists on Fran Visco's extensive mailing list. Visco even allowed Genentech to attach a covering letter, written over her signature, endorsing the trials.

The campaign began to pay off. New enrollments in 648 climbed from fourteen in May 1996 to twenty-one in June and thirty-four in July. Fuchs's effort undoubtedly spurred much of the response by publicizing the open trial slots in the breast-cancer-treatment community. Still, for the most part, enrolling in the trial required the unflagging efforts of the patients themselves. An amazing number eventually fought their way into the trial not because their oncologists had told them about it but because they had read about it on the Internet, heard about it from a friend, or seen a TV or newspaper report.

That is how Anne McNamara, who had spent the better part of two decades fighting breast cancer, finally heard about the treatment that would save her life. In early 1995, she had undergone high-dose chemotherapy and seemed at first to respond. But within three months of completing the treatment, she noticed that two lymph nodes had swollen up again. Scans showed that the cancer had recurred a fourth time. It had spread to several of the lymph nodes in her neck, to her hipbone and collarbones, and to her skin, which had turned red and itchy. "When it was there in the bones, I said to myself, 'This is it.' I knew from reading that that's considered incurable at that point, and I was really depressed," she says. "I was devastated at that point because I figured I had tried everything. It had recurred very quickly. I was trying to decide what to do and thinking this is the first time I ever really thought this is it, I'm not going to make it. I was really depressed."

The ensuing days and months were very difficult, McNamara admits. She was deeply concerned about her husband, Jeff. Luke, their son, was now eighteen years old, and neither she nor Jeff had told him about the cancer. The nights were even harder. She would have trouble going to sleep and would invariably awaken at four in the morning.

And then she had a nightmare that remains emblazoned in her mind. "It was a very symbolic dream," McNamara remembers. "It was so scary that it woke me up. We have a fireplace and a wood-stove, and we light fires and sit around the living room. The fire was burning and I went to put another log on; and it was this big log and it was black and dark. I put the log on and I'm watching it and it starts to burn a little bit and the log turned into the head and body of a black Doberman pinscher. Suddenly he was starting to burn, and he opened his eyes—these yellow, evil eyes. He looked at me, and then he opened his mouth with the teeth as it was burning, as if to say, 'You can't kill me.' It scared the shit out of me, and I woke up in a cold sweat. I think that was a symbol of the cancer that had come back. We tried everything. It wasn't going to die. And it was going to get me."

But on November 5, 1995, she came across an article in *The Boston Globe* with the headline THE DOCTOR IS ON LINE: INTERNET BEING CONSULTED ON HEALTH DATA. The story described how a fifty-year-old women in Shrewsbury, Massachusetts, Karen Caviglia, had used her computer to share her experiences with other cancer patients. More important for Anne McNamara, it told how Caviglia, whose cancer had spread to her bones, had scoured the Internet for information on new treatments and had found out about the Her-2/neu trials then taking place at Boston University Medical Center. McNamara had heard about the antibody a couple of years earlier in conversations on a breast-cancer listserve— an asynchronous conversation over the Internet—but she had dismissed it because it seemed too controversial. Now the article reported that Caviglia had submitted a sample of her tumor, tested positive for the antibody, and was admitted to the trial. In Caviglia's story, McNamara saw a chance for herself.

She got Caviglia's number from directory assistance and phoned her. "I called, but I didn't hold out much hope," she says. "Still, I said to myself, 'If I don't give everything my best shot—if there's anything to be done, you ought to do it. Give it a shot. What have you got to lose?' I'd never forgive myself if there was a chance and I didn't go for it." Caviglia by that time was so sick that she could not start on the new therapy. She gave McNamara the information she needed about the trial. McNamara immediately called Boston University and had her tumor tested. She was Her-2/neu positive.

"It was just dumb luck that [Caviglia] happened to be interviewed in the paper," says McNamara. "Otherwise, I wouldn't have known what was going on." Caviglia never got a chance to start on Her-2/neu; she died within a few months.

In January of 1996, Anne McNamara entered the 649 protocol offering antibody without chemotherapy. Her doctor warned her going in that in some people Her-2/neu stops a tumor's growth but does not make it disappear and in other people the drug has no effect at all. But for Anne the antibody's effect was almost immediate. "The second week after getting the Her-2/neu, I could tell. 'Well,' I thought, 'this is my imagination that my lymph nodes were smaller,' and I said, 'No, no, no—it's just wishful thinking,' " she recalls. "But they really started shrinking right away, and within a month they could not be felt. It was very rapid. The skin involvement started going away after two months. [Then it] was all gone." By the second month, the bone metastasis in her hip had disappeared, and nine months into the protocol the one in her collarbone was only barely visible. "I've been declared a complete response," she says. "And it happened very rapidly," she adds. "So I am just on top of the world. I'm very excited about it. Knowing that the long-term prognosis is not known, but this is the best news I could have had at this point, when I thought there was no news to be had. I was a goner."

Anne McNamara can't help wondering what would have happened to her if she had not come across that newspaper article. She knows her oncologist would probably not have recommended it on his own. The first time she had tried to get into a clinical trial, the one for immune therapy, for which she did not ultimately qualify, her oncologist was enthusiastic about helping her find the right trial. But she had to pursue it. The oncologist she was seeing when she found out about Her-2/neu was less supportive. "He didn't say no. He said it sounded OK to him. But I found it and pursued it and arranged it all on my own."

Referring to herself as "rather an agnostic," McNamara says that over the years she hadn't spent a lot of time in church, even though she and her family are members of one house of worship in town. "I felt I've had to go back to church now," she says, "to thank somebody. *Somebody.* I don't go every week, I go every *other* week," she recounts with a hearty laugh. "My mother would be pleased with that."

These days, McNamara says that she doesn't have trouble sleeping anymore. An avid gardener all of her life, she admits that when her cancer recurred the last time and she thought she was going to die, she saw no point at all in cultivating her garden. "What's the use in that?" she remembers thinking. "I'm enjoying my garden again," she says, breaking into a smile filled with joy, "planting for the future because I think there may be a future."

She worries about patients who are not as plugged in to the online world as she is, because there is such a bounty of information available on the Internet. She also worries about patients who are too timid to challenge their doctors when it comes to their own medical care. "I think patients have to be more active in their own care," she says. She is particularly worried about older women, who are more likely than younger women to regard their doctors as demigods. The women who made their way to the Her-2/neu trial are fighters, unwilling to accept a final negative answer from a doctor.

About the now-deceased Karen Caviglia from Shrewsbury who never had a chance to begin the treatment, McNamara feels terrible. "If she hadn't given that interview in the paper," she says with her customary compassion, "I would never have known about this. I know another woman on the BU program who saw that same article and that's why *she* called. I feel very indebted [to Karen]. I've said prayers for her numerous times. I hope she hears them."

Anne McNamara remembers when she was planning her funeral. "Now I don't think that way anymore. It's still a possibility," she says and then adds, laughing, "It's not in my face, as they say."

———

Fuchs felt he had accomplished his task in jump-starting the Her-2/neu trials. After nine years at Genentech, he quit in August 1996 to take a position with a new biotechnology company, Intrabiotics. He thought it offered him the opportunity to carry out research and clinical trials unfettered by the corporate power struggles he felt often diluted Genentech's efforts. He also received a substantial stake in the company before its initial public stock offering. "California dreamin'," he called it.

Fuchs's job went to Steven Shak, his friend and close colleague who had actually developed Pulmozyme, the cystic fibrosis drug, and had joined Genentech in 1988. A slight, energetic man who wears a mustache and glasses and has an infectious smile, Shak had nothing to do with the Her-2/neu project before he joined it. But Shak proved to be a quick study. Though much more conformist to the corporate culture than Fuchs, he managed to maintain the increasing momentum for the trial that Fuchs had established.

Even with enrollment picking up, Dennis Slamon, whom Fuchs privately had often called Dennis the Menace, was fed up with what he perceived as the glacial speed of testing his drug. He undertook a one-man campaign to expedite the battle plan. He focused on the 649 trial, the one in which Anne McNamara had enrolled, designed for women with metastatic breast cancer who had failed to respond to chemotherapy. All two hundred slots had been filled by September 22, 1996 (222 women ultimately signed up). The protocol called for following the progress of all patients in all the trials for a year, meaning that the results of 649 would be available by September 1997. Observing patients in the trial at UCLA, Slamon believed that the drug was shrinking tumors in enough of them that Genentech could win FDA approval on the basis of the 649 trial alone. Slamon made his case to Genentech and got some measure of sympathy, but in the end he was rebuffed.

On December 9, 1996, he arrived at FDA headquarters in Rockville, Maryland, to tell any FDA officials he could find that a drug that might help thousands of women with breast cancer was languishing as the manufacturer awaited results of one arm of the trial even though it was accumulating results from another arm that it could soon submit. It was a highly unusual move for an individual investigator, but Slamon was determined to accelerate the speed by which the treatment—his treatment—got to women with breast cancer. Through contacts within the FDA, he managed to meet with Susan Jerian, the oncologist already designated to head the review of the Her-2 application, if it ever arrived, and her supervisor, Patricia Keegan. Slamon received a polite but noncommittal response, although he had reason to think his gambit might end up putting the pressure on Genentech.

Michael Friedman sees the FDA as the midwife in drug development. "We're not the parents. We're not the inventor. We're not the producer. We're not the marketer of the product," he explains, "But we're responsible for the birth of that product, and if things don't go well because of a difficult delivery, we're responsible for that. So our job is to make sure that things go as quickly and smoothly as possible." Still, no one doubts that the FDA can pressure drug companies to speed up their efforts in response to political trends.

In fact, in 1995, the Clinton administration was pushing for progress in treating strokes, and a division of the National Institutes of Health had been testing Genentech's heart attack clot discovery, t-PA, as a possible stroke treatment. The company was moving slowly with its request for approval because t-PA can cause bleeding in the brain that can do far more damage than the stroke itself. Nevertheless, the FDA, according to Friedman, "invited" Genentech to work through the 1996 Memorial Day weekend to finalize its application, and on June 18 the FDA was able to announce the approval in record time, only three months after Genentech first filed its preliminary application. The political pressure to bring a breast-cancer drug to market surpassed the pressure for a stroke treatment. If the FDA accepted Slamon's argument that data could be submitted earlier than planned, Genentech would feel the heat.

But Genentech had no desire to submit the results of only the 649 study, which tested the antibody on women who had not responded to one or two rounds of chemotherapy. The company's ultimate goal was to market the antibody as adjuvant therapy for use after surgery. In theory, one quarter or more of the 180,000 women diagnosed with breast cancer every year would be candidates, a huge market. But the company feared it would take even longer to reach this gigantic market if the drug were approved on the basis of a protocol that tested the antibody only on women with advanced metastases. Soon after Slamon visited the FDA, Susan Hellmann, Curd's boss, argued that filing the 649 study might needlessly waste the FDA's time and energy, especially if a second filing for the pivotal 648 study would soon follow. It would be far better, Hellmann said, to "put in an integrated summary of safety and efficacy, one safety package, one efficacy package." Sound logic to be sure, but as long as slots remained open in the 648 trial, which tested the antibody with CA, the harder it would be for Hellmann and other Genentech officials to justify withholding the completed 649 data from the FDA.

Fortunately for Genentech, enrollment continued at a steady pace. In September 1996, forty-two women signed up; in October, fifty-nine; and in November, fifty-five. Word of mouth was a big factor. Anecdotes began to circulate among oncologists about just how good the Her-2/neu antibody could be. Charles Vogel, a Miami oncologist who had helped Genentech plan the trials, remembers "the first four women that I treated did not respond. They all did poorly. Then all of a sudden, I had one, then another, then another—who were responding." Vogel had particularly good results with the 650 trial, for women with newly metastatic breast cancer who refused chemotherapy. "These are women who come in and say, 'I'll never take chemotherapy, but I'll take herbs and roots and this and that,' " Vogel explains. "So I figured that I would at least have something scientific to offer them." In one of Vogel's patients, liver metastases disappeared completely. Another patient had an excellent partial response in liver metastases. Another patient's visible lesion above the collarbone disappeared in four days. "This sort of thing, plus the [responses of women in the other arms of the trial], made me *very* excited about this compound," he says.

Pat Alpert was one of those patients. Alpert had had a mastectomy at age forty-four, and had gone through standard CMF adjuvant chemotherapy. When her cancer recurred five years later, she was flabbergasted at its extent. Blood tests showed her liver enzymes were off the charts. The next step was a series of scans. "I took a friend with me and I went for an ultrasound, a gallbladder ultrasound, which shows the liver as well. And [the radiologist] started marking and marking and marking, tumor after tumor. And I said to him, 'It's very bad, isn't it? Could it be gallstones?' And he said, 'No, this is liver mets.' And I said, 'How long do you think I have?' He said, 'I would go home and make funeral arrangements. You probably have a month.' "

Tumors covered 90 percent of Alpert's liver; additional scans confirmed the cancer had also spread to her lungs and bones. Alpert bought a cemetery plot, videotaped good-bye messages to her friends and relatives, and began a grueling round of chemotherapy for a stem-cell transplant. She also continued to search for information on new treatments. "You can't sit in your room and look at the four walls and expect somebody to knock on your door and say, 'Come and get it.' "

A family friend steered her toward Her-2/neu data and Dr. Vogel. In April 1996, she became one of the first beneficiaries of the compassionate-access program created by Genentech in response to pressure from the activists. Alpert's cancer had failed to respond to many rounds of chemotherapy, making her ineligible for the principal clinical trials. She submitted her name to the lottery and "won" the right to get the antibody.

Alpert's progress was slow at first, but scans a few months after she began treatment revealed that most of her lesions had disappeared. Where she had once felt despair, she is now hopeful. Always active and involved, Alpert now spends much of her time talking with cancer patients, encouraging them and trying to give them hope. "As [the tumors] started to go down and I began seeing other people that had such great results, I made up my mind that I can't sit and worry about dying. That was not living. I started getting involved in different things, and my life is so full now. I never thought it could be as happy and fulfilling as it is."

Such inspiring anecdotes emerged from Europe and Australia and across the United States. To be sure, the treatment did not help every Her-2/neu-positive breast-cancer patient who entered the trial. In some women the antibody accomplished nothing. Others saw their tumors respond for months, only to resume growing. Among the most wrenching outcomes were metastases to the brain. Large molecules the size of the Herceptin molecule seldom cross the blood-brain barrier, so the drug cannot pursue rogue cancer cells that manage to slip into the brain. The doctors talking to one another knew of several women who saw their cancer shrink or disappear from their lungs, livers, and bones, only to spring out as brain tumors.

In the spring of 1997, Kathy Crooks, whose "Andromeda strain" of breast cancer had shrunk so dramatically, thought she was suffering a severe sinus infection. "A lot of symptoms were driving me crazy. I couldn't write my last name. My coordination was off a little bit." Crooks visited Cobleigh for a checkup on Friday, June 13. In the doctor's office she vomited and passed out. Admitted to the hospital, Crooks quickly learned that CT scans revealed metastases in her brain.

The next day technicians administered a huge dose of whole-head radiation. Before the procedure Melody Cobleigh, her doctor, warned of a less than 1 percent chance that her respiration could cease and asked if she wanted to be revived if it happened. Crooks said she did not.

The procedure, however, yielded no life-threatening complications. Crooks took steroids to help reduce brain swelling and went home feeling fine. She remembers the days after the treatment. "It takes a while for the radiation to kick in, and then you *don't* feel fine. You feel absolutely *totally* exhausted. You can't even crawl out of bed." After a few weeks the symptoms subsided, the brain tumors shrank, and Crooks returned to her job and family.

Occasional brain metastases were not the only problem. Earlier that year reports surfaced of a dangerous, unexpected side effect of the Her-2/neu antibody. Back in 1994, as Genentech was planning the phase III trials, John Curd had suggested that the company carry out a quick phase II trial with the combination of antibody and Adriamycin that would make up the principal treatment for the trial. Eager to get moving, Genentech management had vetoed the extra phase II but had instead asked the Data Safety and Monitoring Board, the panel of outside experts that monitors the trial, to take a close look at the first sixty patients taking the combination to check for any unexpected side effects. In September 1996, the board reported to Shak that nothing out of the ordinary seemed to be occurring. A few months later, Shak discovered that the reassurance was premature.

Every day, he scanned what are called adverse-condition reports. Standard trial procedure requires every investigator to report within twenty-four hours every negative, unexpected change in a patient's condition. Looking through the reports in late February 1997, Shak discovered an unusually severe case of cardiac failure in a woman who was taking the antibody in combination with Adriamycin. Progressive weakening of the heart muscle is a common complication of Adriamycin, especially at high doses. But in that report and subsequent ones, Shak saw clear evidence that in some women the antibody could exacerbate this deadly side effect and even trigger it at lower doses. "This wasn't predicted at all on the basis of the preclinical studies," he says. He immediately sent warning letters to the FDA and to every investigator in the study. No one had died—yet—but a handful of women were severely debilitated. No longer could anyone regard Her-2/neu as a drug totally free of side effects. It was a setback that might have been avoided had the company carried out a phase II study that correlated with phase III.

Would the side effect render the drug useless? Was it helping enough women so that it could win FDA approval? Only the final trial results could answer those critical questions. On March 18, 1997, Twaddell, Fuchs, and Shak joined nine veterans of the Her-2 project staff for dinner at the One Market Plaza restaurant in San Francisco to celebrate a milestone: the 648 trial had finally enrolled its goal of 450 women (a total of 469 actually signed up), twenty-two months after Twaddell had first spelled out the protocol and a year after Fuchs had rewritten it. The end was in sight at last. By then, a few women who had initially enrolled in the trial with placebo had been treated for more than a year, and Genentech sent each a dozen roses to mark the occasion. If all continued as planned, Shak would have the 648 results in March 1998.

A few months later, he made a startling calculation: he would have the results of the pivotal 648 trial many months sooner than he had planned. It was the first time in its long odyssey that the new treatment moved faster than anyone had anticipated. The key measure in 648 was what cancer researchers call "time to progression": the interval between the beginning of treatment and the spread of the metastatic cancer. If women taking the antibody escaped a recurrence for a longer time on average than the women taking no antibody, that would prove that the antibody delayed or stopped the cancer growth. When Genentech first planned the 648 trial, it assumed that on average women treated for metastatic breast cancer would suffer a second recurrence nine months after they began treatment. This is the standard assumption, and it shows just how frightening the outlook is for women when their breast cancer returns.

Based on that assumption, the statisticians calculated that the investigators would have to follow all the women in the trial for twelve months to learn whether the antibody offered any meaningful benefit. Shak studied the investigators' reports. While the trial design prevented him from knowing who was getting the antibody and who was not, he could tell that on average all the women in the trial were getting new cancers far more rapidly than anyone had anticipated. Since all the women in the trial were Her-2/neu positive, it turned out to be yet another reminder of the insidious, highly malignant nature of Her-2/neu-positive breast cancers. But it meant that the trial would yield meaningful results much sooner than was planned. The results would be in by early November 1997—five months earlier than anyone had thought. Slamon's effort to force Genentech to submit the 649 data alone now made no sense. All parts of the trial would conclude at about the same time, and Genentech could plan to submit a comprehensive application to the FDA in the spring of 1998. Shak was thrilled with his new discovery. "It was like the room exploded," he said.

With the new results about to come in, Genentech devoted more personnel to the Her-2/neu effort. What had once been a tiny and often neglected part of the company now became its biggest division. By the time the results did arrive in November, two hundred Genentech employees were working full-time on Her-2/neu, and the gloom of failure that had enveloped the effort for so long at last evaporated.

Just before Thanksgiving of 1997, Shak phoned Slamon and told him he had something to share that he could not discuss on the telephone. Slamon remembers his urgent tone. "I didn't know whether to laugh or cry." On the Friday after Thanksgiving, Shak flew to Burbank and in the dark bar of the Burbank Airport Hilton shared the results that Slamon would later call "sensational."

The numbers unequivocally established a position of great importance for Herceptin in the treatment of breast cancer. In the 648 trial far more women remained cancer free with the combination of Herceptin and chemotherapy than those on chemotherapy alone. In the 649 trial the drug shrank or eliminated tumors in significant numbers of patients who had an especially bleak outlook.

With the positive results in hand, Shak, along with other Genentech scientists, flew to Washington to brief Mario Sznol, acting chief of the investigational drug branch at the National Cancer Institute. As central command in America's War on Cancer and with an annual budget of $2.4 billion, the NCI might reasonably be expected to be on top of any positive developments. But the institute had shown little interest in Her-2/neu. In fact, the NCI turned down a grant application from Slamon to study the gene and its application as a cancer treatment in 1989, shortly before he got the money from Revlon. Genentech had kept the NCI at arm's length, fearing that government involvement would only slow its efforts at drug development. Now with the trial successfully completed, Genentech was seeking all manner of help, and the NCI was eager to bask in the glow of success.

Step one was that the NCI agreed to take over the compassionate-access program—supplying the drug prior to FDA approval—through the same lottery system at the nation's thirty-two comprehensive cancer centers and at several military hospitals. Now women seeking the drug through the lottery were being offered a much broader choice of locations. Only once before had the NCI given out a drug through compassionate access, supplying Taxol to women with advanced ovarian cancer from November 1992 to February 1993. Three years after the San Francisco activists had begun their bitter fight to win access to the treatment, the federal government was now actually running the effort.

In order to test drugs, the NCI sponsors several large coopera-
tive networks of oncologists. What Genentech wanted most ur-
gently was for the NCI to sponsor tests of Herceptin as an adjuvant
treatment, to be given to patients soon after surgery. This represented the biggest market of all, and there was good reason to believe that Herceptin, like other cancer treatments, might work far
better were it administered during an earlier stage of the disease.

The NCI contact would prove crucial. But from the instant
Genentech scientists learned of the positive results, the company's
principal task centered on winning FDA approval. "The clock is
ticking," said Bob Cohen, a Genentech oncologist who was assist-
ing in running the effort. "We've got the data, and the FDA cannot
begin their work until they get it."

But preparing the Biological License Application (the BLA, as
the application is formally known) is no simple matter. Genentech
had conducted several large, complicated trials that had generated
enormous amounts of information. The best guess was that there
were twenty thousand pieces of data for each woman who had volunteered for the trials. Of course, the most essential items involved
cancer progression or the lack of it, with or without antibody. But
the overwhelming documentation offered all sorts of other details
gathered about all the women. For instance, when did they first get
breast cancer? Where was that cancer located? What were their risk
factors? When were they initially identified? Were they treated in
the adjuvant setting, and if so, with what? When did they get
metastatic disease? What were they treated with? Which drug?
What dose? When did it start? When did it stop? All the information could help decide what patients would benefit most from the
drug.

In addition to the medical data, Genentech needed to satisfy the
FDA by proving that it could consistently manufacture pure Her-2
antibody in sufficient quantities to meet the expected demand.
Like Genentech's other products—t-PA, human growth hormone,

and Pulmozyme—Herceptin is a large protein that can be manufactured only by growing enormous numbers of genetically identical animal cells (ovary cells from hamsters for Herceptin) in huge vats. Manufacturing requirements for Herceptin would be especially difficult because the dose would be high and women would get the treatment for years, possibly for the rest of their lives.

To carry out the highly specialized production of proteins from cells, Genentech began construction in 1995 of its new plant in Vacaville, forty miles east of San Francisco. For a time, the company imagined it might be able to manufacture Herceptin at the new plant, but construction delays were to change those plans. At the beginning, Genentech would produce Herceptin at its South San Francisco facility, which was already making the company's other products, as well as fourteen experimental compounds at various stages of preliminary trials. According to Cohen, if the demand for Herceptin turned out to be as large as expected, some of the company's other research projects might suffer. "If necessary, if pushed to the wall, we will have to cannibalize other things to make the drug here," Cohen said. And if all went according to plan, Genentech would then alter its submission to the FDA in early 1999, allowing for production to be moved to the new facility at Vacaville.

For its part, the FDA did not sit silently and wait for all the information it needed from Genentech to approve the Her-2/neu drug. In a series of face-to-face and telephone conversations beginning in June 1997 Susan Jerian and her staff members, the FDA officials who would be responsible for the review, met with Genentech representatives to specify exactly what data Genentech would submit and in what form. The FDA did not want to be surprised by any procedural errors that might slow the approval process. In March 1998 Michael Friedman told Genentech that Herceptin had been officially designated to receive fast-track approval. The designation, part of the effort President Clinton had announced in

March 1996, committed the FDA to decide whether to approve the drug within six months of receiving the final application. To expedite the process, Genentech began to submit parts of its application even before it completed the entire effort.

On Friday, May 1, dozens of members of the Her-2 team worked feverishly in the War Room, the center of action in the company's regulatory-affairs division. Gathering together the critical clinical data, they were completing the last part of the submission. Racing to the finish line, they stuffed a seemingly endless pile of folders with the necessary data into boxes, piled the boxes onto hand trucks, and frantically hauled them out to a waiting FedEx truck just ahead of the 5 P.M. deadline for delivery to the East Coast.

It is the moment that all the people working in drug companies live for. Following tradition and to proclaim the achievement, each member of the team struck a bell on the wall outside the War Room. Inside, the mood was celebratory. The team took photographs of one another. They devoured chocolate-covered strawberries. They drank champagne. They listened to congratulatory speeches from Genentech officials, including Art Levinson and Bill Young. In that room, every person who had been part of the Her-2 team knew that medical history was about to be made.

CHAPTER 12

Springtime in L.A.

Two weeks after Genentech sent the data to the FDA, eighteen thousand cancer specialists descended upon the Los Angeles Convention Center for the thirty-fourth annual meeting of the American Society for Clinical Oncology. There was a rare sense of anticipation. The announcement of the Herceptin results would distinguish this as the most newsworthy ASCO meeting in memory. But with so many parents claiming to be responsible for bringing Herceptin into the world, its birth was bound to get complicated. In the City of Angels, tension and jealousy threatened to bedevil the proceedings.

For years, Ronald Perelman and Revlon had remained mostly silent about their contributions to Slamon's research. But in January 1998, Perelman's representative, Jim Conroy, issued a press release that quoted Slamon: "The science that ultimately led to the development of the drug would not have happened when it did without the support of Revlon." Genentech officials did not quite agree. They set out not only to downplay Slamon's involvement but also to put into soft focus all the dissension and delays that had plagued the program for so many years. One of their goals was to get word to the outside world, especially to the investment community, that Herceptin had been the logical result of the solid research and development Genentech carries out all the time. Rational and focused, that is how the company wanted to be perceived.

In an interview in March 1998, CEO Art Levinson had said, "Everything we do here is a controversial project," emphatically maintaining that there was "nothing unusual" about Her-2. Upon hearing Levinson's sentiments, Mike Shepard, who had fought so hard for the project, laughed and imitated a typical Valley Girl with his one-word comment, "WhatEVer!"

Conroy's efforts to publicize Revlon's contributions did not end with the January press release. On Friday, May 15, the day the ASCO delegates began arriving in L.A., the former political operative achieved a public relations triumph. The story he had set up appeared in *The Wall Street Journal*, featuring the cartoon of Slamon with models Cindy Crawford and Halle Berry. The timing was perfect. The article focused mainly on "how a lipstick company thrust itself to the front lines of the War on Cancer," thereby illustrating "a surprising and risky strategy of corporate philanthropy." The piece mentioned Genentech only once, and at that, it was merely in passing. It quoted Perelman as bragging that "there were not a lot of people willing to do this." He went on to say, "If the research wasn't productive, we would've spent money to no avail, but that was a risk we were willing to take."

Corporate sponsorship of cancer research and treatment is hardly novel. In fact, Larry Norton attends patients in the Evelyn M. Lauder Breast Center of Sloan Kettering, named after the matriarch of the Estée Lauder cosmetics fortune. But Perelman, a billionaire who enjoyed his reputation as a ruthless deal maker, seemed to have achieved far more return on his investment than most corporate sponsors. Slamon told the *Journal* the "Revlon grant helped accelerate the research that led to Herceptin by as much as ten years." Even some of Slamon's supporters considered this time line to be somewhat generous. Genentech officials feared the world would believe that the company that created "won't-kiss-off" lipstick developed their breakthrough breast-cancer drug.

Genentech had to fight back.

Revlon's Conroy had rented a small, unassuming booth amid the giant drug-company exhibits in the convention's commercial area. Revlon representatives handed out modest pamphlets explaining the company's effort and clipboards labeled REVLON/UCLA WOMEN'S CANCER PROGRAM. On Saturday, just before Genentech's planned press conference at a nearby hotel, Conroy left a stack of the pamphlets and clipboards in the convention's pressroom for the fifty or so reporters who were covering the meeting.

Paul Laland, Genentech's smooth-talking director of corporate communications, openly ordered Conroy to remove the material.

"How can you tell me what to do in a space that's not yours?" retorted the indignant Conroy, displaying his feistiest New York Irish street-fighting attitude. Laland apparently did not want Revlon diluting his company's crucial moment. He said Revlon's press release contained inaccuracies, a charge Conroy denied. Eventually, with Slamon's intervention, the brouhaha ended and the two men reached a compromise: Conroy would not replenish his pile of materials until after the press conference. Conroy left in disgust, and Slamon was more furious than ever at Genentech. "I've had it with these people," he said tersely.

Despite his irritation, Slamon played the role of the stalwart trouper at Genentech's press conference that Saturday afternoon, arranged to brief reporters twenty-four hours before the formal conference presentations. As if the strained atmosphere was not already at the point of snapping, the drab, tiny Malibu B room in the basement of the Grand Hyatt Hotel was hot enough to keep everyone drenched in sweat. Most of the key players in the Her-2 saga sat facing three rows of reporters and cameras positioned a mere ten feet away. Susan Hellmann and Steve Shak from Genentech, with Slamon, Melody Cobleigh, Debu Tripathey, Fran Visco, and

Charles Vogel, all shared the podium. Larry Norton would arrive later.

Hellmann spoke first, followed by Shak. Like many companies, Genentech sends key employees for media training, but Shak was clearly in need of a refresher course. He appeared almost too nervous to open his mouth, and concluded his prepared remarks with pat phrases obviously minted in the PR office: "Herceptin is another example of the promise of biotechnology fulfilled. Herceptin is a sparkling jewel of Genentech science."

Slamon was next. In an understated way, probably for the thousandth time in his career, he recited the history of the Her-2 project, beginning with the observation that the concept of "throwing bigger and better bombs" at breast cancer "wasn't going to get us a whole lot further." He detailed the 648 data. Cobleigh followed with the 649 results. Then Visco spoke, praising Genentech's cooperation with the National Breast Cancer Coalition, while carefully avoiding a direct endorsement of the drug. She emphasized her long-standing campaign to bring more patients into clinical trials. Noting that only 3 percent of adult cancer patients take part in trials, she said, "If that number does not go up we will not be having many more press conferences like this one." As she was speaking, Norton hustled into the room. Visco introduced him, and he quickly took his place at the podium.

Norton told the reporters there was "no question" the drug would be used widely as soon as it was approved. He said much bigger studies could now get under way. In fact, he said, he was helping plan these studies that very afternoon. "That's why I came late and why I'll have to leave early," he explained. The moment was his.

Slamon could barely maintain his composure. Now Larry Norton had not only found profound faith in Herceptin, he was leading the congregation. After his urgent last-minute arrival from Herceptin-trial-planning conferences, he was taking charge. To make matters worse, when Slamon had spoken about the data, he had been vigilant in his attempt to remain responsible and to add all the qualifiers. Even when he managed to say, "We're excited by these results," his tone was so restrained that he sounded almost sleepy, making it hard to believe he meant it. Norton, on the other hand, offered forceful sound bites. "This is the biggest difference I've ever seen in a trial of advanced breast cancer," he proclaimed with absolute conviction. "Nobody that I know of has ever seen a trial where the two arms are that different." Because of his impassioned presentation, it was Norton who appeared in most of the subsequent news reports about Herceptin. Readers or viewers might easily conclude that Larry Norton had developed Herceptin. In the final tally Slamon and his Revlon-sponsored network had enrolled forty-three women in the critical 648 trial. Norton enrolled two.

Drug companies work hard to be kind to oncologists. That evening, Johnson & Johnson invited all the physicians at ASCO to a dinner and a private performance by *Tonight Show* host Jay Leno. Slamon decided to skip the festivities. Jumping into his Nissan 300ZX, he picked up Jim Conroy at the Peninsula Hotel and managed to get a rare Saturday night reservation at Chinois on Main in Santa Monica to rehash the day's frustrations.

Finally, on Sunday afternoon, the ASCO delegates heard the results. The convention runs from Saturday morning through Tuesday, scheduled on a weekend so that busy physicians can return as quickly as possible to their practices. Typically, the most important presentation takes place late afternoon Sunday and the delegates— almost all eighteen thousand of them—packed into the session titled "Her-2/neu in Breast Cancer."

Drug companies almost never designate their own scientists to present important trial results. They choose academics who confer the aura of independent respectability. Even though Genentech officials regarded Slamon as a pit bull to be trusted only occasionally, they had no choice but to offer him the role of presenting the key 648 data. The company asked Melody Cobleigh, the mild-mannered oncologist who had treated Kathy Crooks, to detail the 649 results. Three speakers preceded her, and then it was Cobleigh's turn.

Cobleigh was terrified. She had never addressed an audience even a tenth as big as this one. Her husband had surprised her by flying in with their two sons from Chicago to watch her big moment; and their presence, while welcome, only heightened her anxiety. But in soft-spoken tones, she offered a presentation that electrified the assembled cancer specialists. The oncologists were all too familiar with the type of patients who made up the volunteers in 649. The women had undergone initial treatment when their cancers first struck—surgery often followed by radiation and adjuvant therapy. But then their cancers returned and refused to succumb to chemotherapy. George Sledge, Jr., a breast cancer expert from Indiana University who would speak at another session of the meeting, called attempts to treat such women "a graveyard, both metaphorically and literally."

But Cobleigh offered solid evidence that Herceptin could help women with seemingly intractable metastatic breast cancer. Two hundred thirteen patients completed the study. Eight had achieved a "complete response"—their cancer disappeared. Twenty-six had a partial response, with their tumors shrinking by 50 percent or more. As precisely measured by the independent-response-evaluation committee, these were the most reliable numbers—the "squeaky-clean" data the FDA would consider. But Cobleigh pointed out that the investigators themselves thought Herceptin was much better than that. In at least 30 percent of the women, she said, the tumors did not shrink; neither, though, did they grow. These women were listed officially as not having benefited from the treatments. But such stability could well be the goal of relatively nontoxic therapies of the future.

Cobleigh also noted that among the women in the study whose cancer had failed to respond to the biggest cannon of all—high-dose chemotherapy with bone-marrow rescue—more than one quarter benefited significantly from Herceptin. The responses persisted on average for 9.1 months, hardly an eternity. But Cobleigh said she found that amount of time to be "especially gratifying." Her audience clearly agreed.

As Cobleigh continued her talk, there was a subtle but noticeable change in mood. When she began, she was like many investigators at this meeting, factually and simply detailing the results of a study. But after ten minutes or so, it was resoundingly evident that she was going further, filling in her colleagues on the clinical features of a new treatment they all soon would be offering.

She addressed the matter of the fever and flulike symptoms that struck about 40 percent of the patients after they received their first infusion. "Let me talk heart to heart to the clinicians," she said. "Your nurse is going to come running and say to you that this patient looks lousy. And you will go see the patient and you will agree. But relax." Cobleigh explained that in most cases a dose of the painkiller Tylenol and the antihistamine Benadryl would quickly solve the problem, which almost never occurs after the first infusion. She pointed out, to the continuing amazement of even the most experienced of these cancer specialists, that often the positive responses "occurred very rapidly."

Without mentioning names, Cobleigh told the story of Kathy Crook's astonishing and instantaneous return from the precipice of death. It was an anecdote that impressed even the most cynical in this army of cancer-treating veterans. At the end of most medical-meeting presentations, the audience offers scattered and polite applause. When Melody Cobleigh finished, the applause was thunderous and sustained.

Then it was Slamon's turn. While Cobleigh's presentation was a smooth description of a medical triumph, Slamon took some time to tell his version of the history of Her-2 and to settle some scores. It was a highly unusual start to the presentation of data from a major clinical trial. At one point, he talked about how he and his team decided "to move this drug" into clinical trials, adding—after a long pause—"in collaboration with Genentech." Reminding everyone that the effort had begun in his own laboratory, he showed a slide from his 1987 *Science* paper, depicting the very same gel that his undergraduate student, Wendy Levin, had used to discover that Axel Ullrich's Her-2/neu gene was overexpressed in some breast tumors. This research, he said, made the gene "a logical target" for therapy. He further reminded the audience that Genentech's antibody was not the only one he tested. He went back over his discovery that cisplatin and the antibody worked better together than either alone—the effect was "synergistic"—whereas the chemotherapy drugs actually used in the trial, Adriamycin and Taxol, were merely "additive" to Herceptin and thus inferior. Undercutting the very results he presented, he told the audience, "I don't know that we had the best combination of drugs."

Despite these caveats, the results of the crucial 648 trial, combining Herceptin with chemotherapy, remained impressive. Herceptin together with other chemotherapy drugs, such as cisplatin, might indeed work better, and future clinical trials would determine that. But the combinations used in this trial worked quite well enough to bring Herceptin to clinical practice. The trial measured several things. One was "time to progression"—how long after treatment began before the cancer started to grow again. When added to chemotherapy, Herceptin increased that interval by 65 percent, from 4.6 months on average to 7.6 months.

Another key measure was how much the women's tumors shrank. Forty-nine percent of the women taking Herceptin with chemotherapy saw half or more of their cancer disappear. Only 32 percent of the women taking chemotherapy alone had the same response. The most dramatic effect of Herceptin was in combination with Taxol. Taxol, the most powerful breast cancer drug available, shrank tumors in only 16 percent of the women. But when Herceptin was added to the Taxol, the response nearly tripled to 40 percent.

The one serious side effect of Herceptin appeared to be the cardiac toxicity, first noted by Shak. It struck 13 percent of patients who got Herceptin in the trials, compared to 4 percent who did not get the antibody. But since the complication occurred mostly in women who were being treated or had been treated with Adriamycin, doctors would know how to guard against the side effect in the future, and would be able to treat it when it did strike.

Even more than the results that Cobleigh had just presented, the 648 numbers offered incontrovertible evidence that Herceptin would quickly find a crucial place in the care of women with breast cancer. At the end of his talk, Slamon barely thanked the Genentech scientists, but he did offer extensive appreciation to Revlon and to Jim Conroy; to Mike Shepard, "who stuck by this program through thick and thin"; and to Hank Fuchs, who "got this trial on track."

That evening, Genentech hosted cocktails and dinner at the Hollywood Terrace, an outdoor café at the peak of a hill in the middle of the Universal Studios lot in North Hollywood. The company invited all the investigators, as well as most of Genentech's Her-2 team. The activists came too: Marilyn McGregor and Bob Erwin from San Francisco, and Fran Visco from the National Breast Cancer Coalition. It was a spectacularly clear evening. The warm orange glow of the setting sun over the San Fernando Valley set the tone of the festivities. Everyone at this party could celebrate an enormous success. Women's lives would be saved, and a huge fortune would be made.

The one person conspicuous by his absence was Dennis Slamon.

Epilogue

Ginger Empey

As Slamon and Cobleigh were presenting the phase III Herceptin results, Ginger Empey, the youthful-looking nurse who was the first to enroll in those very trials, watched from an aisle of the packed convention center auditorium. She searched for Steve Shak, whom she had seen in a television report, and the others from Genentech. "I looked so hard for people. I really tried to find people I wanted to touch base with, to thank them, and, you know, acknowledge everything, and I couldn't find anybody. There were only eighteen thousand people there!" She laughs, recalling the scene. "It was the biggest room I've ever seen in my life. You could have dropped two football fields down the middle of that room and not even touched the sides!"

Empey, who was marking her one hundred forty-third week on the drug, had emerged as something of a Herceptin media star. She had appeared in several newspaper and magazine articles and on TV programs about the drug's success. "Isn't it a hoot?" she enthusiastically asked. "This is one of the things I prayed for that summer when I was waiting to get the antibody: one, that I would *get* the antibody; two, that the antibody would work; and three, that I would be the poster girl for the drug!" Just being able to stand there among scientists and doctors, most of whom well understood the deadly prognosis she had received three years ago, was a thrill: "It was like, *I am alive! I am here!*"

The UCLA press office had asked her to appear at the Genentech press conference on Saturday, but then retracted the invitation. Slamon had vetoed the idea because he felt that her presence might have shifted the focus away from the science, and toward the high emotion of Empey's escape from imminent death. Empey made her way to the conference on her own anyway, thanks to the generosity of cousins in Pacific Palisades who knew how much she wanted to be there. They wrote her a check for most of the $450 registration fee. If they hadn't, Empey would not have been able to witness this moment: the unfolding of the scientific history she had helped to create.

Several times during various media interviews, Empey said she thought Herceptin was a miracle. Reporters were skeptical, but Empey was steadfast. "When I think of all this stuff coming together, it was pretty darn close to a miracle. When you have a certain faith and miracles are part of that, then this is a big one. According to my belief system, this is big stuff."

Kathy Crooks

Watching the news coverage of Herceptin from her home in Illinois, Kathy Crooks, the feminist and industrial supplies business owner, experienced a mixture of emotions. Herceptin had saved her life, as Cobleigh had told it, when Crooks was literally hours from dying. Certainly Crooks was amazed at how lucky she was. "Heck," she remarked, "two months later I was out swimming in the ocean, and I should have been dead!" Yet Crooks worried that too many women with breast cancer would get the idea that Herceptin is the ultimate cure. "People don't realize that only a certain small percentage are going to qualify to take the drug... and only a percentage of that will do well on it." Crooks knew from experience that even the most dramatic responses did not always last.

Even though she continued her weekly infusions of Herceptin, Crooks was struggling to stay healthy. After having recovered in early 1997 from whole-head radiation to treat the cancer that had spread to her brain, she suffered another setback. CAT scans in December of that year revealed that the cancer was roaring back, invading her lungs, liver, and the bones of her lower back. Cobleigh, her doctor, decided to try not an entirely new approach, but the one Dennis Slamon had tested in phase II trials: adding cisplatin to the Herceptin. It was the combination of drugs that had saved Barbara Bradfield, and was the one Dennis Slamon had fought so hard and unsuccessfully to include in phase III.

For several months, Cobleigh had been experimenting with Herceptin and cisplatin in women whose cancer failed to respond to Herceptin alone. She was impressed with what she saw. "Phenomenal results. It looks like Slamon was right from the beginning." Indeed, Slamon as well as other scientists were already planning to conduct studies of the combination now that Herceptin was on its way to FDA approval.

Crooks became terribly sick from cisplatin. "Nothing gets accomplished," she said. "You might have one day of the week where you're functioning." The four months of misery turned out to be worth it. By the time of the ASCO conference in May, she was once again cancer free. The metastases to her liver, lungs, and bones had amazingly disappeared. Still, Crooks thinks she would be kidding herself if she were to believe that the cancer was gone for good. "That's being a fool, in my opinion. I know that this is like riding a roller coaster. It goes up. It goes down. It goes up and goes down. This is what's going on."

Although she is the ultimate realist, Crooks firmly believes when the drug is approved, Herceptin is going to make an enormous difference. "If all the other physicians can network to get this information and can start doing it within the next six months, think of all the families that'll have Mom around to go through adolescence with their children." Crooks is one of those moms. Her own son, Devin, was eight years old and was with her at her appointment when she first learned she had breast cancer. She had comforted the crying boy, saying, "I just have to take my medicine and I'll be fine." At the time, she had no idea how life-threatening her cancer was, nor how complicated taking her medicine would become.

Just recently, Devin, now an adolescent, asked her to teach him how to slow dance. "That was such a sweet thing," she says, softly. "To be able to be here and have those experiences, to think through that, that I wouldn't be here if it weren't for Herceptin, there's no doubt in my mind that thousands of women could have these same stories. Just to give them more quality time, just to see things, and prepare for things, and not be sick—that is critical."

Crooks fully expects to survive well into old age. "I think my eyes will do me in, to be honest!" she says. But coping with cancer's chronicity keeps daily life in perspective. "You have to look at life as the short time we're on the planet, and it's a gift. And we forget that. When I look at the sky and I see those beautiful clouds, it means a lot more to me than it does to someone else that doesn't have cancer."

Barbara Bradfield

Barbara Bradfield, who owes her life to the Herceptin-cisplatin combination, approached her sixth cancer-free year with a mixture of wonder and concern. "It's thrilling," she said, "and sad, too, because of all the ones that didn't make it." On that Sunday afternoon of the big presentations in the L.A. Convention Center, John Dreyfuss, head of media relations for UCLA's Jonsson Cancer Center, had called her to tell her everything was going fine, and that "Dennis was the star."

As the longest survivor of all, Bradfield has appeared often in news reports about Herceptin. As the drug has made its laborious way through the required trials, she has frequently been in the spotlight. She has been glad to share her experience. But doing so had brought an unanticipated consequence. "I get phone calls every week from people, desperate people, who have picked my name out of an article or something," she says, thoughtfully, "and it's been frustrating because there wasn't any [clinical trial] they could get into." The expected approval of Herceptin will make her job easier. "At least now it's going to be possible to tell them what to do and what to ask for, and they'll be able to get it."

Trying to help the women with breast cancer who regularly contact her has only reinforced Bradfield's abiding distrust of the medical profession, the skepticism she acquired after her own diagnosis. She encourages women who contact her to ask their doctors questions. "One disturbing thing that I have come up against is that so many doctors are so close-minded. And arrogant. And they won't listen to their patients about something new. I had one girl who actually was tested for Her-2/neu, and the doctor talked her out of trying to get into the trial." When asked what she believes is the thinking behind this behavior, Bradfield says matter-of-factly, "Money, money, money. I'm convinced." Doctors, she says, don't want to lose the income every patient brings in. She carefully excludes Dennis Slamon from this group. "He's been very wonderful.

"For me, it's been a big education, because I was one of those who thought that doctors all loved their patients and had their best interests at heart," Bradfield says. "I never would have believed all this if I hadn't experienced it myself."

Pat Alpert

Pat Alpert has also learned through her battle with breast cancer not to trust most doctors, even though she is married to one. She considers her husband to be an exception. She and many of the women in the trials believe that it was solely their own research and self-advocacy that led them to a cutting-edge drug like Herceptin, and that only their own efforts will continue to help them. "I can't expect that my doctor is going to be my one source of knowledge," Alpert says. "If I want to stay alive, I have to do my homework." Her husband helps her search the Internet for new information.

Like Empey and Bradfield, Alpert has appeared on television and in newspaper stories many times in the Miami area because of her positive response to Herceptin. People seek her out for advice. Additionally, because of her volunteer work acting as a hospital liaison with cancer patients, Alpert sees a lot of desperate situations and hears many stories that infuriate her. She thinks doctors don't tell their patients about new cancer treatments until it's too late. "They either don't know any better because they're not keeping up and they don't know what's going on, or because financially they don't want to lose the patient," she says. "I've seen it over and over again."

As the ASCO meeting was taking place, Alpert was involved in researching her next treatment. She continued to take Herceptin, but blood tests and a CAT scan showed a tiny spot of breast cancer on her liver. Yet she felt fine physically. "You just have to stay one step ahead," she said, adding, "you just have to stay alive long enough" until better treatments come along.

Alpert saw Lilly Tartikoff on the *Today* program and decided to write her a letter, "to tell her how much I appreciate what she's done in giving me the last two years of my life."

Mary Bonesco

Mary Bonesco of Brooklyn has now passed the five-year mark, cancer free. She and her husband, Vince, continue their weekly routine of driving to Manhattan to Sloan Kettering. "It's part of life and I've learned to deal with it, and every Friday, it's hospital day." Always practical, Mary sees the FDA's approval of Herceptin as something that might loosen up restrictions on where and how she gets her infusions. "I want to see if I can make it a little easier on myself," she says. "Have an infusion closer to the house, even have a nurse come in."

As things now stand, Vince must work late four nights a week to make up for the time he takes off each Friday to drive Mary into New York. And being absent every Friday has prevented Mary from getting a better job at the day-care center where she works. To make matters worse, neither the Bonescos' insurance nor Genentech's clinical trial paid the accumulating cost of care at Sloan Kettering, putting a financial drain on the couple's income.

For five years Mary has never missed an infusion. At one point, her brothers and sisters were considering a family trip to Italy. Her original doctor, José Baselga, had returned to the University of Barcelona and could have given her an infusion there if she traveled to Europe. But Bonesco decided it was not worth the effort. "Why," she asked, "would I want to take a chance, take a gamble with my life, staying away from something that's keeping me alive?"

Anne McNamara

Anne McNamara had been taking weekly infusions for more than two years at the time of the ASCO conference and had had an excellent response. But battling breast cancer for two decades had tempered her hopes about Herceptin. "I've been going through this for twenty years now, with numerous recurrences. So I tried not to let myself think of it as a cure."

Sure enough, some cancer did recur in May 1997, after she had been on Herceptin for a year. McNamara suffers from lymphedema, a swelling in the arm on the side of her mastectomy. It is a common and lasting side effect of the surgery, caused by the severing of crucial blood vessels as well as the vessels that transport white blood cells in the lymphatic system. Sores emerged on her swollen upper arm. She soon discovered them to be mounds of breast cancer cells. "I am distressed by all this, but not devastated," she said at the time. "I have done so well that I am hopeful this can be managed."

Ever analytical, McNamara reasoned that the cancer appeared on her arm because poor blood circulation, due to the lymphedema, prevented the Herceptin from reaching the site. She asked the doctor treating her in the clinical trial to consider injecting Herceptin directly into the lesions. Her doctor refused because it would violate Genentech's FDA-approved protocol. McNamara then called other trial investigators to ask their opinion. She was gratified to learn they thought it was an intriguing idea. Ultimately, though, she was frustrated that they, too, refused to violate protocol.

By early 1998, Anne was feeling restless. The cancerous sores not only remained but were "slowly getting a little larger, spreading out, like a puddle." She didn't like thinking about what they were doing. "There are cancer cells there," she said, pointedly, "and some of them are no doubt breaking off and going to the rest of the body." She was fairly certain that the Herceptin was keeping them from growing elsewhere, but she wanted to get rid of them. Back on the Internet, using a combination of search terms like "intralesional" and "cutaneous," McNamara discovered a paper written by a retired physician at Columbia-Presbyterian Medical Center in New York. "It was like a beacon there," she says. The emeritus professor Luciano Ozzello had successfully treated such skin tumors with a combination of alpha and gamma interferon. Interestingly, these were two of the drugs that once failed to work against most cancer in Genentech's clinical trials in the 1980s but were still available. McNamara wrote Ozzello a letter describing her situation, and he sent her reprints of his published papers as well as details of his unpublished work.

With those papers in hand, McNamara went back to her oncologist, who "was impressed," but still would not provide injections. Once again taking matters into her own hands, McNamara worked out an arrangement with her family-practice doctor and a local dermatologist to write her a prescription for the interferons. She injected the drugs herself. Within a few weeks, the menacing skin lesions shrank, and a subsequent biopsy showed no sign of cancer cells.

McNamara was looking forward to seeing her oncologist a few weeks after the ASCO meeting for a routine checkup. "I haven't seen her in about four months, and she hasn't seen the results," she says. With unusual immodesty, she adds, "I'm going to go show her, and wave the biopsy in front of her and gloat."

Twenty years of confronting breast-cancer recurrences has taught McNamara well. She knows how to watch out for herself and to be realistic about treatments. But even she is awed by her experience with Herceptin.

"My response to it, I think, is just miraculous," she says. "I'm still agog at how well it has worked out for me, that I just kind of stumbled into it, and it's just made all the difference in the world. I marvel at that. Why me? What does the future hold? Who knows? There are new discoveries popping up every day, so maybe something more in the curative line, I'll live to see. I hope."

NOTES

When I was a graduate student at the University of California, Berkeley, in the late 1960s, I tinkered with antibodies in an attempt to treat cancer. Those experiments in mice were wildly unsuccessful. I soon switched to a career in science journalism. But I offer the anecdote to demonstrate the length of my interest in the topic of designing better means of treating cancer, especially using elements of the immune system.

This is a work of journalism based mostly on my interviews and observations. The principal interview subjects are listed below, along with other sources and references.

The inspiration for this project sprang from several reports for the *NBC Nightly News, Today,* and *Dateline NBC* that I prepared beginning in April 1996. In addition to the specific interviews conducted for the book, I have drawn on the reporting for those programs as well as on much of my other coverage of biomedical research over the past twenty-five years.

Interview Subjects

VOLUNTEERS FOR THE HERCEPTIN TRIALS

Pat Alpert
Mary Bonesco*

* Identity disguised at the subject's request.

Barbara Bradfield
Susan Brook
Kathy Crooks
Nina Davids
Ginger Empey
Anne McNamara*
Edith Sooy

OTHERS (listed with current institutional affiliations)

Karen Antman, Columbia-Presbyterian Medical Center
David Baltimore, California Institute of Technology
José Baselga, University of Barcelona
Barry Bloom, Albert Einstein Medical College
David Botstein, Stanford University
Melody Cobleigh, Rush-Presbyterian-St. Luke's Medical Center
Robert Cohen, Genentech
Steven Come, Beth Israel, Boston
Jim Conroy, MacAndrews and Forbes
John Curd, Genentech
Bob Erwin, Biosource Technologies
Nancy Evans, Breast Cancer Action, San Francisco
Michael Friedman, Food and Drug Administration
Hank Fuchs, Intrabiotics
Jeff Getty, ACT-UP/Golden Gate
John Glaspy, UCLA
Daniel Hayes, Georgetown University
Susan Hellmann, Genentech
Craig Henderson, Sequus Pharmaceuticals
John Kennedy, Johns Hopkins
Mary-Claire King, University of Washington
Laura Leber, Genentech
Philip Leder, Harvard Medical School

Art Levinson, Genentech
Dan Maneval, Canji Pharmaceuticals
Ron Martell, Genentech
Marilyn McGregor, ACT-UP/Golden Gate
Robert Moulton
Larry Norton, Memorial Sloan Kettering Cancer Center
James Ntambi, University of Wisconsin
Mark Pegram, UCLA
William Peters, Karmanos Cancer Institute
Joseph Schlessinger, New York University
Lynn Schuchter, University of Pennsylvania
Steven Shak, Genentech
Mike Shepard, New Biotics
Dennis Slamon, UCLA
Mark Slikowski, Genentech
Lilly Tartikoff
Robert Temple, Food and Drug Administration
Debu Tripathey, University of California, San Francisco
Tom Twaddell, Otsuka America Pharmaceuticals
Axel Ullrich, Max Planck Institute, Munich
Charles Vogel, Columbia Cancer Care
Frances Visco, National Breast Cancer Coalition
Robert Weinberg, Massachusetts Institute of Technology
Janet Wolter, Rush-Presbyterian-St. Luke's Medical Center
Bill Young, Genentech

And a few who wished to remain anonymous.

Sources

1. Discovering Cancer

6   The National Cancer Institute mailed letters to thirteen thousand
     oncologists during the week of May 13, 1988, alerting them to

three then-unpublished clinical trials demonstrating an increased survival in breast-cancer patients undergoing adjuvant treatment.

7 The odds of a thirty-two-year-old woman being diagnosed were supplied by Brenda Edwards, National Cancer Institute, personal communication.

10 For more on the perception of cancer as a women's disease and for an excellent history of cancer in America, see James T. Patterson, *The Dread Disease, Cancer and Modern American Culture* (Cambridge: Harvard University Press, 1987).

11 Current death-rate figures are from *SEER Cancer Statistics Review 1973–1995* (Bethesda, MD: National Institutes of Health, National Cancer Institute, 1998). Numbers from 1950 were provided in a personal communication by Brenda Edwards of the NCI.

11 Roswell Park quoted in Patterson, *The Dread Disease.*

11 Historical budget figures for the National Cancer Institute were provided by the National Cancer Institute office of public affairs.

12 *"never...confuse cancer research"*: Robert A. Weinberg, *Racing to the Beginning of the Road: The Search for the Origin of Cancer* (New York: HarperCollins, 1996). This book offers a fascinating and detailed popular account of cancer research in the 1970s and 1980s. For the more technical version, see Robert A. Weinberg (ed.), *Oncogenes and the Molecular Origins of Cancer* (Cold Spring Harbor Laboratory Press, 1990).

12 For details of ancient cancers see Michael R. Zimmerman, "An Experimental Study of Mummification Pertinent to the Antiquity of Cancer," *Cancer* 40 (1977), pp. 1358–62.

13 *"answers to the cancer problem"*: Weinberg, *Racing to the Beginning of the Road.*

2. A LIMITED ARSENAL

21 For a history of the beginnings of radiation therapy, see Nancy Knight and J. Frank Wilson, "The Early Years of Radiation Therapy," in *A History of the Radiological Sciences: Radiation Oncology,*

Raymond A. Gagliardi and Wilson J. Frank (eds.) (Reston, Va.: Radiological Centennial, Inc., 1996).

22 Five-year survival rates: See Patterson, *The Dread Disease,* and John Bailar II and Elaine Smith, "Progress Against Cancer?" *The New England Journal of Medicine* 314 (May 8, 1986), pp. 1226–32.

22 For accounts of the sinking of U.S.S. *John Harvey* and its place in the development of chemotherapy see Kevin Coughlin, "Mustard Gas a Weapon so Horrible even Hitler Refused to Employ It," The Newark (N.J.) *Star-Ledger,* November 10, 1995, and Beth Harpaz, "War Gas Leak Was Hushed Up," The Northern New Jersey *Record,* May 29, 1988.

23 For accounts of the secret tests carried out on U.S. personnel, see Tony Freemantle, "The Price of Peace: A Painful Past / Blisters and Lies / World War II Navy Guinea Pig Kept the Dark Secret for Nearly 50 Years, Even from His Wife," *Houston Chronicle,* November 23, 1997; Gary Warner, "The Secret Mustard Gas Experiments, Accidents in WW II, Thousands Ordered to Breathe Diluted Forms to Test Uniforms' or Equipment's Ability to Withstand Chemicals," *Orange County Register,* March 8, 1993; and William Ruberry, "Secrecy Is Lifted on War-Gas Tests," *Richmond Times-Dispatch,* March 11, 1993.

24 *"penicillin for cancer":* The New York Times, October 3, 1953, cited in Patterson, *The Dread Disease.*

24 Details on drugs from "Antineoplastic Agents for Breast Cancer," Gold Standard Multimedia, 1998.

25 *"only the beginning of cancer":* Aulus Cornelius Celsus, *De Medicina,* cited in Roberta Altman, *Waking Up Fighting Back: the Politics of Breast Cancer* (New York: Little, Brown, 1996).

25 For a history of hormone treatment, see V. Craig Jordan, *Tamoxifen: A Guide for Clinicians and Patients* (Huntington, NY: PRR, 1996).

27 The National Cancer Institute presented the tamoxifen prevention results at a press conference on April 13, 1998. The two-year raloxifene results were presented at the ASCO meeting on May 18, 1998. As of this writing, publication of both studies is pending.

3. A New Way of Doing Science

30   For an excellent account of the early years of Genentech, including Ullrich's role, see Stephen Hall, *Invisible Frontiers: The Race to Synthesize the Human Gene* (New York: Atlantic Monthly Press, 1987).

33   A. Ullrich, L. Coussens, J. S. Hayflick, T. J. Dull, A. Gray, A. W. Tam, J. Lee, Y. Yarden, T. A. Libermann, J. Schlessinger, J. Downward, E. L. V. Mayes, N. Whittle, M. D. Waterfield, and P. H. Seeburg, *Nature* 309 (1984), pp. 418–25.

34   Two other groups (that both used the term erb-b-2) cloned the gene at about the same time as Ullrich's. The references are: L. Coussens, T. L. Yang-Feng, Y. C. Liao, E. Chen, A. Gray, J. Mc-Grath, P. H. Seeburg, T. A. Libermann, J. Schlessinger, U. Francke, A. Levinson, and A. Ullrich, "Tyrosine Kinase Receptor with Extensive Homology to EGF Receptor Shares Chromosomal Location with neu Oncogene," *Science* 230 (1985), pp. 1132–39; T. Yamamoto, S. Ikawa, T. Akiyama, K. Semba, N. Nomura, N. Miyajima, T. Saito, and K. Toyoshima, "Similarity of Protein Encoded by the Human c-erb-B-2 Gene to Epidermal Growth Factor Receptor," *Nature* 319 (1986), pp. 230–34; C. R. King, M. H. Kraus, and S. A. Aaronson, "Amplification of a Novel v-erbB-related Gene in a Human Mammary Carcinoma," *Science* 229 (1985), pp. 974–76.

40   D. J. Slamon, G. M. Clark, S. Wong, W. J. Levin, A. Ullrich, and W. L. McGuire, "Human Breast Cancer: Correlation of Relapse and Survival with Amplification of the Her-2/neu Oncogene," *Science* 235 (1987), pp. 177–82.

41   D. J. Slamon, W. Godolphin, L. A. Jones, J. A. Holt, S. G. Wong, D. E. Keith, W. J. Levin, S. G. Stuart, A. Udove, A. Ullrich, and M. F. Press, "Studies of the Her-2/neu Proto-oncogene in Human Breast and Ovarian Cancer," *Science* 244 (1989), pp. 707–12.

45   *"We... always had fun"*: Charles McCoy, "Genentech's New CEO Seeks Clean Slate," *The Wall Street Journal*, July 12, 1995. Accounts of Genentech's questionable marketing practices include that article and Joan Rigdon, "U.S. Is Widening Probe of Genentech

Drug's Marketing," *The Wall Street Journal*, July 11, 1995; Carl T. Hall, "Genentech Executive Forced Out Questions About Leadership, Ethics," *San Francisco Chronicle*, July 11, 1995; Lawrence M. Fisher, "Rehabilitation of a Biotech Pioneer," *The New York Times*, May 8, 1994; Marylin Chase, "Battle of Heart Attack Drugs Heats Up," *The Wall Street Journal*, March 8, 1990; and Marylin Chase, "Lost Euphoria, Genentech Battered by Great Expectations Is Tightening Its Belt," *The Wall Street Journal*, October 11, 1986.

46   Quotes from Krim are from Robert Teitelman, *Gene Dreams: Wall Street, Academia, and the Rise of Biotechnology* (New York: Basic Books, 1989), an excellent account of the fervor over interferons and the role of Mathilda Krim.

4. Courting the Thought Leader

54   For details of the Roche buyout of Genentech, see Joan O'C. Hamilton, Linda Jereski, and Joseph Weber, "Why Genentech Ditched the Dream of Independence," *Business Week*, February 19, 1990.

58   Linda Marsa, "One Last Chance: Ovarian Cancer Is Killing Diane Hinton. Conventional Treatments Have Failed. Now Her Life Depends on an Experimental Therapy That Would Block the Action of a Deadly Gene," *Los Angeles Times*, October 20, 1991.

7. The Mayor of the Infusion Room

88   "*when you die at ninety-five*": Susan M. Love and Karen Kindsey, *Dr. Susan Love's Breast Book* (New York: Random House, 1995). This is by far the best single source for women and their families seeking information about breast-cancer treatment.

90   "*the first one hundred patients*": Carey Quan Gelernter, "A Pioneering Life," *The Seattle Times*, October 15, 1990.

9. TRIALS AND ERRORS

135 ABC News *20/20* carried an excellent report on the allegations about stock options on March 8, 1991.

11. STRAWBERRIES AND CHAMPAGNE

152 Regarding Raab's departure from Genentech, see Charles McCoy, "Genentech's New CEO Seeks Clean Slate," *The Wall Street Journal*, July 12, 1995, and Carl T. Hall, "Genentech Executive Forced Out Questions About Leadership, Ethics," *San Francisco Chronicle*, July 11, 1995.

156 Regarding Genentech's relationship with the FDA in seeking approval for t-PA, see Michael Specter, "Rejection of Heart Drug Was by the Book; FDA Demand for More Information on Safety of Clot-Dissolver Was Unexpected," *The Washington Post*, September 13, 1987, and Joan O'C. Hamilton, "Birth of a Blockbuster: How Genentech Delivered the Goods," *Business Week*, November 30, 1987.

161 For details of Genentech's growth hormone marketing, see Werth Barry, "How Short Is Too Short?" *The New York Times*, June 16, 1991.

INDEX

ABOUT THE AUTHOR

ROBERT BAZELL is the chief science correspondent for NBC News. His reports, which appear on the *NBC Nightly News, Today,* and *Dateline NBC,* have won every major award in broadcasting. He has written for many publications including *The New Republic, The New York Times,* and *The New York Review of Books.* He lives in New York with his wife, Margot, and daughter, Stephanie.

ABOUT THE TYPE

The text of this book was set in Janson, a misnamed typeface designed in about 1690 by Nicholas Kis, a Hungarian in Amsterdam. In 1919 the matrices became the property of the Stempel Foundry in Frankfurt. It is an old-style book face of excellent clarity and sharpness. Janson serifs are concave and splayed; the contrast between thick and thin strokes is marked.

DATE DUE

Demco, Inc. 38-293